MIX
Papier aus verantwortungsvollen Quellen
Paper from responsible sources
FSC® C105338

Dana R. Mohammed

Photographical Analysis of Macro- and Micro-aesthetic Appearance

A Cross-Sectional Study of Iraqi Adults with Class I Normal Occlusion

Anchor Academic Publishing

Mohammed, Dana R.: Photographical Analysis of Macro- and Micro-aesthetic Appearance. A Cross-Sectional Study of Iraqi Adults with Class I Normal Occlusion, Hamburg, Anchor Academic Publishing 2018

Buch-ISBN: 978-3-96067-202-9
PDF-eBook-ISBN: 978-3-96067-702-4
Druck/Herstellung: Anchor Academic Publishing, Hamburg, 2018
Covermotiv: © Designed by Freepik

Bibliografische Information der Deutschen Nationalbibliothek:
Die Deutsche Nationalbibliothek verzeichnet diese Publikation in der Deutschen Nationalbibliografie; detaillierte bibliografische Daten sind im Internet über http://dnb.d-nb.de abrufbar.

Bibliographical Information of the German National Library:
The German National Library lists this publication in the German National Bibliography. Detailed bibliographic data can be found at: http://dnb.d-nb.de

All rights reserved. This publication may not be reproduced, stored in a retrieval system or transmitted, in any form or by any means, electronic, mechanical, photocopying, recording or otherwise, without the prior permission of the publishers.

Das Werk einschließlich aller seiner Teile ist urheberrechtlich geschützt. Jede Verwertung außerhalb der Grenzen des Urheberrechtsgesetzes ist ohne Zustimmung des Verlages unzulässig und strafbar. Dies gilt insbesondere für Vervielfältigungen, Übersetzungen, Mikroverfilmungen und die Einspeicherung und Bearbeitung in elektronischen Systemen.

Die Wiedergabe von Gebrauchsnamen, Handelsnamen, Warenbezeichnungen usw. in diesem Werk berechtigt auch ohne besondere Kennzeichnung nicht zu der Annahme, dass solche Namen im Sinne der Warenzeichen- und Markenschutz-Gesetzgebung als frei zu betrachten wären und daher von jedermann benutzt werden dürften.

Die Informationen in diesem Werk wurden mit Sorgfalt erarbeitet. Dennoch können Fehler nicht vollständig ausgeschlossen werden und die Diplomica Verlag GmbH, die Autoren oder Übersetzer übernehmen keine juristische Verantwortung oder irgendeine Haftung für evtl. verbliebene fehlerhafte Angaben und deren Folgen.

Alle Rechte vorbehalten

© Anchor Academic Publishing, Imprint der Diplomica Verlag GmbH
Hermannstal 119k, 22119 Hamburg
http://www.diplomica-verlag.de, Hamburg 2018
Printed in Germany

Dedication

To My Heaven on Earth "My Beloved Parents": Thank you for your unconditional love that encourages & motivates me to set a higher targets.

Acknowledgement

First of all, immeasurable thanks and praises to "ALLAH" for guiding me and giving me the ambition, willingness and patience to start and complete this work.

I would like to express my gratitude to the post Dean of the College of Dentistry, University of Baghdad, **Prof. Dr. Nabeel Abdul Fatah**, for offering me the opportunity to perform my study.

My sincere thanks to **Dr. Saif Seham Saleem**, the post director of the postgraduate studies, College of Dentistry, University of Baghdad.

My deepest gratitude goes to **Prof. Dr. Nidhal H. Ghaib**, the post Chairman of Orthodontic Department for her kindness, endless help and support during my study, and for all the scientific advices and practical hints she granted us in the practical and theoretical course of the study.

I offer my greatest thanks and sincere appreciation to my supervisor Assist. **Prof. Dr.Iman I. Al-Sheakli**, for her love, care, warm-heartedness and considering me as her daughter, I am grateful for her support, guidance, advices, valuble comments and suggestions that benefited me in completion and success of my work.

My respect and gratitude to our teaching staff of the orthodontic department for their kindness, valuable advices and scientific notes.

I would like to express my appreciation to **Assist. Prof. Dr. Mohammed Nahidh,** for sharing his knowledge, effort, time, valuable advices and enhancing my self-confidence in clinical course, and for helping me in performing the statistical analysis of my study.

My thanks extended to **Mustafa Dhaher** who is a student at College of Art, University of Baghdad, Cinema and T.V Department for helping me in my work, and to all dental students who participated in this study, thank you for your spirit help.

List of contents

Subjects	Page No.
List of contents	1
List of tables	5
List of figures	6
List of abbreviations	9
Abstract	10
Introduction	12
Aims of the study	14
Chapter One: Review of Literature	
1.1. Aesthetics	15
1.1.1. Facial Aesthetics: Art and History	16
1.1.1.a. Pre-Renaissance Period "Toward Body Measurements"	16
1.1.1.b. Renaissance Period "Toward Ideal Facial Proportions and Measurements"	18
1.1.2. Aesthetic Appearance	22
1.1.2.1. Dental-Facial Aesthetics	22
1.1.2.2. Classification of Aesthetic Appearance	23
1.1.3. Facial Beauty and Attractiveness	24
1.1.3.1. Perceptions of Facial Attractivness	24
1.1.3.2. Distinguishing Features	27
1.1.3.3. Social Importance of Facial Aesthetics	28
1.1.4. Soft Tissue of the Face	28
1.1.4.1. Soft Tissue Changes with Growth	28
1.1.4.2. The Nose	29
1.1.4.3. The Lips	30
1.1.4.4. The Chin	31
1.1.4.5. Height and Width of the Face	32
1.2. The Dentition	33
1.2.1. Normal Occlusion	33
1.2.2. Dental Aesthetics	35
1.2.2.1. Dental Aesthetics and Maxillary Anterior Teeth	37

List of contents

1.2.3. Dentofacial Relationships	42
1.3. Methods of Facial Measurements	45
1.3.1. Direct Methods	45
1.3.1.a. Craniometry	45
1.3.1.b. Anthropometry	46
1.3.2. Indirect Methods	47
1.3.2.a. Cephalometric Analysis	47
1.3.2.b. Photographical Analysis	47
1.3.2.c. Three-Dimensional Imaging Analysis	51
1.3.2.d. Cone-Beam Computer Tomography Analysis	52
1.3.2.e. Video-Imaging Analysis	53
1.4. Previous Studies Related to photographical analysis of the facial and dental measurements in Baghdad	53
Chapter Two: Materials and Methods	
2.1. Materials	54
2.1.1. Sample	54
2.1.1.1. Criteria for Subject Selection	54
2.1.2. Instruments and Equipments	55
2.2. Methods	59
2.2.1. Ethical Consideration	59
2.2.2. Clinical Examination	59
2.2.2.1 History	59
2.2.2.2. Skeletal Examination	59
2.2.2.3. Dental Examination	61
2.2.3. Standardization of the Photographs	62
2.2.4. Photographic Exposure	64
2.2.5. The Digital Camera Set-Up	64
2.2.6. Photographic Analysis	65
2.2.6.1. The Macro-aesthetic Appearance	66
2.2.6.2. The Micro-aesthetic Appearance	69
2.3. Pilot Study	72
2.4. Statistical Analysis	75

List of contents

Chapter Three: Results	
3.1. Sample	76
3.2. Descriptive Statistics and Gender Differences in Macro-aesthetic Appearance	76
3.3. Descriptive Statistics and Gender Differences in Maxillary Anterior Teeth Variables	78
3.4. Descriptive Statistics and Gender Differences in Micro-aesthetic Appearance	80
3.5. Descriptive Statistics and Side Difference in Micro-aesthetic Appearance in Male Group	82
3.6. Descriptive Statistics and Side Difference in Micro-aesthetic Appearance in Female Group	84
3.7. Correlation between the Facial Measurements and (mesiodistal width of both central incisors, inter-incisal distance, inter-canine distance, combined mesiodistal width of six anterior teeth) in Male Group	86
3.8. Correlation between the Facial Measurements and (mesiodistal width of both central incisors, inter-incisal distance, inter-canine distance, combined mesiodistal width of six anterior teeth) in Female Group	87
3.9. Correlation Between Mesiodistal Width of each Tooth and the Facial Measurements in Male Group	88
3.10. Correlation Between Mesiodistal Width of each Tooth and the Facial Measurements in Female Group	90
Chapter Four: Discussion	
4.1. Sample	93
4.2. Descriptive Statistics and Gender Differences in Macro-aesthetic Appearance	94
4.3. Descriptive Statistics and Gender Differences in Maxillary Anterior Teeth Variables	94
4.4. Descriptive Statistics and Gender Differences in Micro-esthetic Appearance	96
4.5. Descriptive Statistics and Side Difference in Micro-aesthetic Appearance in Male and Female Group	98

4.6. Correlation between the Facial Measurements and (mesiodistal width of both central incisors, inter-incisal distance, inter-canine distance, combined mesiodistal width of six anterior teeth) in Male and Female Group	99
4.7. Correlation Between Mesiodistal Width of each Tooth and the Facial Measurements in Male and Female Group	100
4.8. Clinical Consideration	103
Chapter Five: Conclusions and suggestions	
5.1. Conclusions	105
References	**106**
Appendices	
Appendix I	136
Appendix II	137

List of tables

Table No.	Table title	Page No.
Table 2.1.	Inter-examiner calibration of the facial measurements	73
Table 2.2.	Inter-examiner calibration of intraoral measurements	73
Table 2.3.	Intra-examiner calibration of the facial measurements	74
Table 2.4.	Intra-examiner calibration of intraoral measurements	74
Table 3.1.	The sample of this study and their mean age	76
Table 3.2.	Descriptive statistics and gender differences in macro-aesthetic appearance for male and female groups	77
Table 3.3.	Descriptive statistics and gender differences in Maxillary anterior teeth variables	78
Table 3.4.	Descriptive statistics and gender differences in micro-aesthetic appearance	80
Table 3.5.	Descriptive statistics and side difference in micro-aesthetic appearance in male group	82
Table 3.6.	Descriptive statistics and side difference in micro-aesthetic appearance in female group	84
Table 3.7.	Correlation between the facial measurements and (mesiodistal width of both central incisors, inter-incisal distance, inter-canine distance, combined mesiodistal width of six anterior teeth) in male group	86
Table 3.8.	Correlation between the facial measurements and (mesiodistal width of both central incisors, inter-incisal distance, inter-canine distance, combined mesiodistal width of six anterior teeth) in female group	88
Table 3.9.	Correlation between mesiodistal width of each tooth and the facial measurements in male group	90
Table 3.10.	Correlation between mesiodistal width of each tooth and the facial measurements in female group	92

List of figures

Figure No.	Figure title	Page No.
Fig 1.1	Queen Nefertiti. The famous face is well proportioned and symmetrical	16
Fig 1.2	Human figures were drawn standing with head and legs in a lateral view and shoulders in the anterior view	17
Fig 1.3	According to Da Vinci, in a well-proportioned face, the size of mouth equals the distance between the parting of lips and the edge of chin	19
Fig 1.4	Two beautiful faces that show the divine proportion of external configuration	20
Fig 1.5	The golden-ratio proportions of the ideal face	21
Fig 1.6	Classification of Aesthetic Appearance	24
Fig 1.7	Nasal growth, pink coloured area shows growth between 10-13 years of age; red coloured area shows growth between 13-16 years of age	30
Fig 1.8	Soft tissue landmarks and horizontal variables for measuring the thickness of the upper lip and soft tissue chin	32
Fig 1.9	Frontal and lateral views of an ideal occlusion	33
Fig 1.10	Angle classification, Facial profile and molar relationship	34
Fig 1.11	Ideal tooth width proportions when viewed from the front	36
Fig 1.12	Preston's proportion	37
Fig 1.13	Height-width proportions for maxillary central incisors	38
Fig 1.14	Golden percentage	39
Fig 1.15	Ideal heights of contact points	41
Fig 1.16	Height of the contact points	41
Fig 1.17	Horizontal facial dimension	44
Fig 1.18	Apparatus used for craniometry devised in 1902	45
Fig 1.19	Anthropometric analysis for facial measurements	46
Fig 1.20	Facial photograph	50
Fig 1.21	Intra-oral photographs	51
Fig 1.22	Stereophotogrammetry with two different coplanar planes for 3D Images	52

List of figures

Fig 2.1	Instruments used in the study	56
Fig 2.2	(A): A digital camera (Canon EOS 60D), (B): (18-200) Lens	57
Fig 2.3	Height adjustable tripod	57
Fig 2.4	Ruler for intraoral photograph	58
Fig 2.5	Ruler for extraoral photograph	58
Fig 2.6	(A): Cephalostat, (B): Blue background, (C): Stool	58
Fig 2.7	Assessment of anteroposterior relation by using Foster method	60
Fig 2.8	Measurement of upper and lower anterior facial heights	60
Fig 2.9	The camera fixed in position with a height adjustable tripod	63
Fig 2.10	The distance between the subjects and the camera lens measured with measuring tap	63
Fig 2.11	The distance between the subjects and the camera lens was 56 cm for intraoral photograph and 101 cm for extraoral photograph	63
Fig 2.12	Participant was positioned in the cephalostat and instructed to look at the center of the camera's lens during taking the photograph	65
Fig 2.13	Facial Landmarks	67
Fig 2.14	The Linear Facial Measurements	68
Fig 2.15	Vertical Facial Measurements	69
Fig 2.16	Measurement of mesiodistal width of maxillary anterior teeth	70
Fig 2.17	Measurement of the height of maxillary central incisors, height of contact points and total maxillary anterior teeth width	72
Fig 3.1	Descriptive statistics and gender differences in macro-aesthetic appearance for male and female groups	77
Fig 3.2	Descriptive statistics and gender differences in Maxillary anterior teeth variables.	79
Fig 3.3	Descriptive statistics and gender differences in micro-aesthetic appearance.	81

Fig 3.4	Descriptive statistics and side difference in micro-aesthetic appearance in male group	83
Fig 3.5	Descriptive statistics and side difference in micro-aesthetic appearance in female group	85

List of abbreviations

ʼ	Soft tissue
%	Percentage
(Θ)	Phi
AutoCad	Auto Computer Aided Design
B.C	Before Christ
Ca	Canine
CI	Central incisor
CIs	Both central incisors
cm	Centimeter
CMDW	Combined mesiodistal width
d.f	Degree of freedom
Fig	Figure
HS	Highly significant
ICaD	Inter-canine distance
IID	Inter-incisal distance
LI	Lateral incisor
MDW	Mesiodistal width
mm	Millimeter
N	Number
NS	Non-significant
P	Probability value
R	Pearson coefficient
S	Significant
SD	Standard deviation
SPSS	Statistical package for social sciences

Abstract

Generally, the facial aesthetics depends on the aesthetic appearance of the maxillary anterior teeth. The aims of this study were to analyse the macro-aesthetic appearance of the face and micro-aesthetic appearance of the maxillary anterior teeth to establish a normative values for class I skeletal and dental relation and investigate the relationship between facial measurements and width of maxillary anterior teeth and mesiodistal width of each maxillary anterior tooth.

The sample consisted of 120 Iraqi adults dental students (60 males and 60 females) with an age ranged between 18-23 years. Each individual was clinically examined according to the specific criteria. The photographic records were taken with cephalostat based head position, frontal facial and intraoral photographic records were performed for each subject by using digital camera that fixed in position with height adjustable tripod; the facial (five horizontal and four vertical distances) and dental measurements were measured by using AutoCad program 2014.

Descriptive statistics were obtained for facial and dental measurements, the mean values were generally higher in males than in females for facial and dental variables, whereas the independent samples t-test showed a high significant gender difference in most of facial variables, and a non-significant gender difference in most of dental variables, additionally, there was a non-significant side difference in most of the measured dental variables in male group, and significant side difference in most of the measured dental variables in female group. Pearson's correlation coefficient was obtained to test the relation between the facial and dental measurements, a non-significant correlation was obtained between most of the measured facial and dental variables.

The present study found that the gender differences were significant in macro-aesthetic appearance (facial measurements) with males having larger facial measurements than females, while the gender had a non-significant effect on the micro-aesthetic appearance (maxillary anterior teeth proportions), on the other hand asymmetry between the right and left side was found in most of the dental measurements, and weak correlation was obtained generally between facial and dental measurements.

Introduction

Mouth and eyes are the most visible structures of a human face and they have a significant importance in formation of someone's personality **(Baldwin, 1980)**, while some authors consider mouth to be even more important than the eye **(Terry and Davis, 1976)**.

It had been recognized for some time that facial beauty was directly affected by the harmonious facial proportions, while this was an intuitive statement for most aesthetic surgeons, now a day an objective data exists to support these conceptual frameworks, *Farkas* and others introduced anthropometric data that used most frequently to determine the ideal facial proportions **(Farkas, 1994)**.

Lombardi in 1973 was the first one who introduced the importance of dental proportions and documented that there was a recurring ratio between all the teeth in relation to the face from maxillary central incisor to maxillary first premolar **(Ward, 2001; Gurel, 2003)**. An interesting division of aesthetics in orthodontics was presented by **Sarver and Ackerman (2005)**, who divided aesthetics into three sections: 1) Micro-aesthetics: which includes the dental aspect, 2) Mini-aesthetics: which includes smile aesthetics, and 3) Macro-aesthetics: which refers to the face, its proportions and harmony.

One of the most important factors in the planning of any orthodontic treatment and assessment of the treatment changes was to evaluate and assess soft tissue first **(Frankel and Frankel, 1988)**.

Evaluation of the soft tissue had been carried out by the means of different methods of evaluation **(Saxena and Thoke, 2012)**, direct anthropometry had several restrictions as a method of clinical documentation or evaluation of facial soft tissue, this technique was limited to the direct measurement of the linear distances between facial landmarks and subjected to operator errors from a different degrees of deformation of the soft tissue by direct contact of the instruments, additionally, a standard lateral cephalometric films had been used to diagnose, provide treatment plan and to predict soft tissue and hard tissue responses to orthodontic treatment, the major limitation of the cephalometry was that the facial soft tissues from the frontal view was not possible to be evaluated **(Holdaway, 1983; Michiels and Tourne, 1990)**.

Two-dimensional photogrammetric analysis had the benefit of being a basic, non-invasive, cost-effective and quick method that required minimal time and equipments in the assessment of soft tissue, most of the studies regarding facial soft tissue evaluation on standardized two-dimensional and life-sized photographs reported the comparison and assessment of racial characteristics, the treatment changes, and differences between genders **(Saxena and Thoke, 2012)**.

Many studies tried to relate the mesiodistal dimension of central incisors or the maxillary anterior teeth to transverse facial measurements in order to get benefit in the selection of artificial teeth for complete dentures **(Scandrett *et al.*, 1982)**. In orthodontics, facial aesthetic is not concentrated on the teeth or jaws separately, but it involves dental and maxillofacial portions **(Ahmed *et al.*, 2013)**.

Although there were Iraqi studies used the photographic analysis of the face; the uniqueness of this study comes from that it is the first study that analyse the micro-aesthetic appearance to establish a normative values for Iraqi population and find out if there is a correlation between apperant mesiodistal measurements of maxillary anterior teeth and facial measurements "by indirect method of measurement by using photographs" in a sample of Iraqi population.

Aims of the study

The present study aimed to:
1. Analyse the macro-aesthetic appearance of the face and micro-aesthetic appearance of maxillary anterior teeth to establish a normative values for Iraqi adults with class I normal occlusion by using photographs and computer analysis.
2. Detect possible gender differences in macro- and micro-aesthetic appearance and possible side differences in micro-aesthetic appearance.
3. Investigate the relationship between facial measurements and mesiodistal width of maxillary anterior teeth.

Chapter One
Review of Literature

"Beautiful is that which pleases universally without a concept"

Immanuel Kant in 1790 **(Naini *et al.*, 2006).**

1.1. Aesthetics

Beauty can be defined as a combination of qualities that gives pleasure to the senses or to the mind, it is a philosophical concept and the aspects of which were studied under the term aesthetics obtained from the Greek word for perception *(aisthesis)* and was coined by the 18th century philosopher *Alexander Baumgarten* who established the aesthetics as a separate field of philosophy, therefore; aesthetics is the study of the beauty and to a lesser extent it's opposite to the term ugly, it involves both the understanding and the evaluation of beauty, proportions and the symmetry **(Naini *et al.*, 2006).**

Facial beauty is a mystery, a complex concept for which there is no equation, or numbers can successfully describe it **(Peck and Peck, 1970; Adamson *et al.*, 2006).**

Facial beauty is easier to recognize than to understand **(Baig, 2004).** Scholars and scientists from time immemorial had studied and tried to understand and explain this complex multifaceted concept **(Barker and Barker, 2002).**

The perception of beauty exists on a subconscious level, when viewing something beautiful, reward centers located in the primitive human brain were activated, facial aesthetics follows the evolutionary and artistic principles of attraction, symmetrical and average faces with balanced proportions were considered to be the most aesthetic, this is harmonious even across cultures, where values and preferences may be significantly different; an attractive person from one culture is likely to be recognized as attractive in a totally different culture **(Collins, 2012).**

CHAPTER ONE

Review of Literature

1.1.1. Facial Aesthetics: Art and History

Greater attention to details, especially of the human face, was recorded by the ancient Egyptian, Greek and Roman civilizations **(Vegter and Hage, 2001)**. The portrayal of the human faces and art through the ages were intricately linked, documented art of the early civilizations served as the medium through which figurations of the ideal facial form and proportion of that time were recorded, these early representations of the human form date back to pre-historic man's rock paintings and stone carvings, art of the Paleolithic era some 35000 years ago showed a poor and infrequent representation of the human form compared with the more numerous and detailed drawings of hunting themes **(Peck and Peck, 1970)**.

1.1.1.a. Pre-Renaissance Period "Toward Body Measurements"

About 5000 years ago, Egyptian civilization marked the first sign of facial beauty displayed in their art works **(Peck and Peck, 1970)**. The most famous painted limestone character of Queen Nefertiti (1350 BC) **(Fig 1.1)**, with her harmonious facial proportions and symmetry, is an example of how the Egyptians immortalized the beauty of their kings and queens by depicting them; the name Nefertiti literally means the *"Perfect One"*. **(Naini and Gill, 2008).**

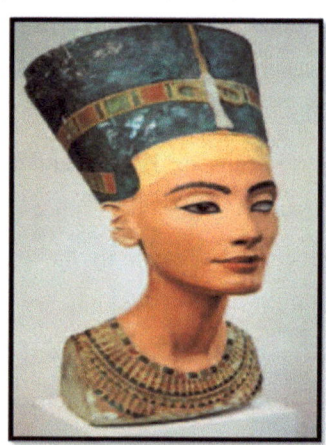

Figure 1.1: Queen Nefertiti. The famous face is well proportioned and symmetrical, (Berlin Museum) **(Naini and Gill, 2008).**

The ancient Egyptians were the first to attempt description of facial and bodily proportions in mathematical form, Egyptian artisans drew human figures as we still know them today, standing with head and legs in a lateral view and shoulders in the anterior view **(Smith *et al.*, 1998; Vegter and Hage, 2000)** as shown in (**Fig 1.2**).

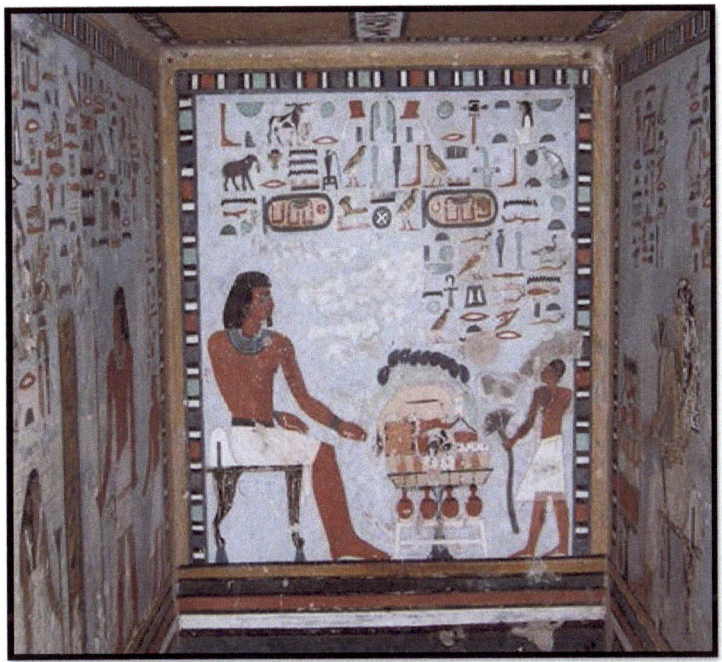

Figure 1.2: Human figures were drawn standing with head and legs in a lateral view and shoulders in the anterior view (Smith *et al.*, 1998).

A Greek sculptor *Polycleitus* (450-420 BC) was obsessed with the beauty of the male athletic bodies, even though Polycleitus study of the ideal physical proportions were probably based on the Egyptian principles, Polycleitus reported that the height of the face was one-tenth of the length of the body and the whole head was one-eighth of the length of the body, head and neck together were to be one-sixth of the length of the athlete **(Snijder, 1928)**.

The Greek philosopher *Aristotle* (384-322 BC) defined beauty as an imprecise sense of a harmonious or aesthetically pleasing proportionality (Aristotle, 1094; **Prokopakis *et al*., 2013)**. Aristotle emphasized the proportions of aesthetics and part of very extensive work of Aristotle dealt with the human body, he proved that certain groups of people appeared to be superior to others, in Aristotle Physiognomica, he described the science of reading one's character from one's bodily features **(Heinemann, 1963)**. Aristotle compared male and female bodies and faces to those of various animals and from this comparison, he found males to look like a brave lions because of the squarer face, square forehead, larger mouth, equally balanced jaws, bright, deep-set eyes and large eyebrows, whereas women in his opinion were more like shy panthers (Aristoteles, 1949; **Vegter and Hage, 2000)**.

1.1.1.b. Renaissance Period "Toward Ideal Facial Proportions and Measurements"

Leonardo Da Vinci (1452-1519) excelled as a painter, sculptor, in addition to architecture, engineering, human physiology and anatomy **(Pedretti, 2001)**. Da Vinci reported on the proportions according to which the bodies and the faces should be ideally shaped, according to Da Vinci, in a well-proportioned face, the size of mouth was equal to the distance between the parting of lips and edge of the chin, while the distance from chin to the nostrils, from nostrils to the eyebrows, and from eyebrows to the hairline were all equal, and the height of the ears was equal to the length of the nose as shown in **(Fig 1.3)**, Da Vinci could not deny the variations of the nature, he did his measurements on the live bodies and compared the sizes of the various parts of these live bodies to one another (McMurrich, 1930; **McCurdy, 1954; Vegter and Hage, 2000)**.

CHAPTER ONE

Review of Literature

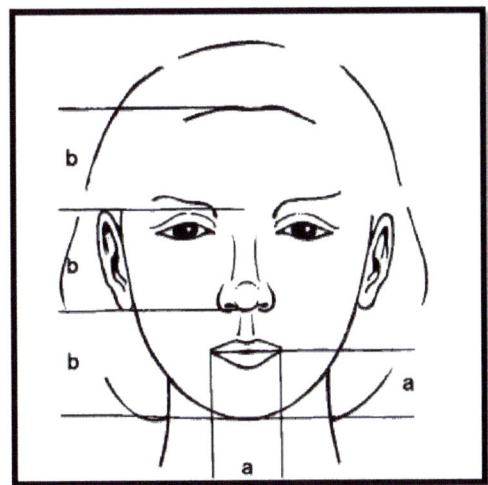

Figure 1.3: According to Da Vinci, in a well-proportioned face, the size of mouth equals the distance between the parting of lips and the edge of chin (a), while the distance from chin to the nostrils, from nostrils to the eyebrows, and from eyebrows to the hairline were all equal (b), and the height of the ears were equal to the length of the nose **(Vegter and Hage, 2000).**

Cesare Lombroso (1836-1909) described how murderers, gangsters, fire raisers, alcoholics, epileptics, and dwarfs could be distinguished from "normal" people by anthropometric assessment and evaluation of asymmetry of the face, shape of the skull, tooth form, shape of nostrils, size of masseter muscle, and size of frontal sinus (Lombroso, 1890**; Vegter and Hage, 2000).**

Ricketts was the first who claimed that the analysis of a physically beautiful faces should be achieved mathematically, and he claimed to use the golden proportions in that respect, *Ricketts* invisualized dozens of photographs of the magazine models to select pairs of distances or measurements that representing a golden proportion in those beautiful faces **(Ricketts, 1982a; Ricketts, 1982b; Jefferson, 2004)** as shown in **(Fig 1.4).**

CHAPTER ONE

Review of Literature

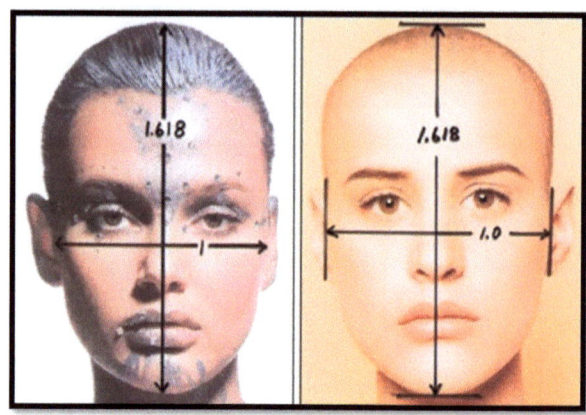

Figure 1.4: Two beautiful faces that show the divine proportion of external configuration **(Jefferson, 2004).**

Ricketts's articles appeared to be the key publications in oral surgery and orthodontics for facial aesthetics **(Ricketts, 1982a; Ricketts, 1982b).** *Ricketts* performed a small study using a ten beautiful faces and defined a several golden proportions in them **(Sinclair, 1982).** *Ricketts* popularized the concept of the "golden proportion" that introduced by *Seghers* in facial surgery, and by using a golden divider *Ricketts* proved that the harmonious faces of the beautiful women were to be built according to the golden proportions *"the ratio that is most attractive to the human eye and mind"* and the Greek letter phi (Θ) was used to indicate the number 1.618, the golden divider was a sliding caliper with which any given distance could be divided in accordance to the 1:1.618 ratio, for example, in some of vertical relationships of the face, if the distance from lateral side of the nose to the soft tissue menton was 1, then the distance from the lateral side of the nose to Trichion (beginning of the forehead wrinkling when one lifts the eyebrow) is 1.618, and if the distance from chilion (corner of the mouth) to the soft tissue menton was 1, then the distance from lateral canthus of the eyes to chilion is 1.618, **(Fig 1.5A)**, additionally, transverse relationships of the face must conform to the golden proportion, for example, if the distance between lateral side of the nose was 1, then the distance between chilion is 1.618, the distance between the lateral canthus of the eyes is $(1.618)^2$ and the distance between the temporal soft tissues of the eyebrow level is $(1.618)^3$, **(Fig 1.5B)**, also the external dimension of adult head must conform to the golden proportion, ideally, if the distance from lateral border of the cheeks was 1, then the distance from top of the head to soft tissue menton should be 1.618, **(Fig 1.5C)**, applying the concept of the golden proportion for planning and evaluating treatment in daily practice has been advocated **(Seghers *et al.*, 1964; Ricketts, 1968; Levin, 1978; Ricketts, 1981; Ricketts, 1982a; Ricketts, 1982b; Jefferson, 2004; Premkumar, 2011).**

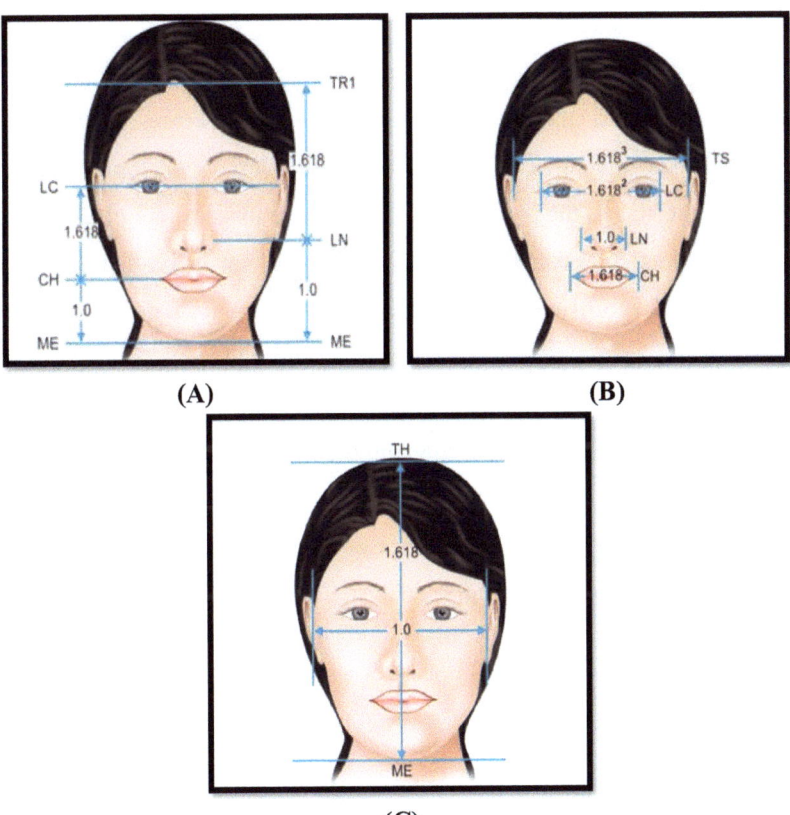

Figure 1.5: The golden-ratio proportions of the ideal face, (A): vertical proportion, (B): transverse proportion, (C): external proportion (Premkumar, 2011).

Farkas considered to be the one who influenced the modern facial soft tissue anthropometry, by measuring and comparing more than 100 dimensions and proportions in hundreds of people, *Farkas* defined a standards for almost every soft tissue measurement in the head and face of more than 120 publications, additionally, *Farkas* explained the role of anthropometric measurements in the evaluation of lateral facial dysplasia and cleft lip and palate **(Farkas *et al.*, 1977; Farkas, 1987; Farkas *et al.*, 1993; Farkas, 1994).**

1.1.2. Aesthetic Appearance
1.1.2.1. Dental-Facial Aesthetics
Dental and facial aesthetics could be defined in three ways:

- **Traditionally,** macro and micro elements terms could represent the facial and dental aesthetics, macro-aesthetics includes the interrelationships between face, lips, gingiva, teeth and the perception that these relationships are pleasing, whereas the micro-aesthetics encompasses the aesthetics of an individual tooth and the perception that the form and the color are pleasing **(Maclaren and Culp, 2013).**
- **Historically,** accepted smile, smile design concepts and smile parameters assist to design aesthetic treatments, these specific measurements of form, color and tooth-aesthetic elements help in transferring smile design information between dentists, ceramists and patients; however, aesthetics in dentistry could include a broad area known as *"the aesthetic zone"* **(Maclaren and Tran, 2009).**
- **Rufenacht** categorized the smile analysis into facial aesthetics, dentofacial aesthetics and dental aesthetics that included the macro and micro elements **(Rufenacht, 2000).**

1.1.2.2. Classification of Aesthetic Appearance

As shown in **(Fig 1.6)**, aesthetic appearance could be classified into:

A- Macro-aesthetics consideration includes: **(Sarver, 2011; Brandão and Brandão, 2013)**

i. Vertical proportions.
ii. Profile.
iii. Lip fullness.
iv. Chin projections, nasal projections, big ears, etc.

B- Mini-aesthetics consideration includes: **(Brandão and Brandão, 2013; Katti *et al.*, 2013)**

i. Smile arc.
ii. Smile types.
iii. Buccal corridors.

C- Micro-aesthetics consideration includes: **(Brandão and Brandão, 2013; Katti *et al.*, 2013)**

i. Tooth proportions.
ii. Tooth shade and color.
iii. Connectors area and embrasures.
iv. Gingival height, shape and contours.

Macro, mini and micro-aesthetics in orthodontics are the considerations that carried out during and at the end of orthodontic treatment to enhance the cosmetic appearance of the patient **(Proffit *et al*, 2007)**.

In addition to previous classification, another classification identifies five levels of aesthetics which include: *facial, oral-facial, oral, dentogingival and dental* **(Maclaren and Rifkin, 2002; Maclaren and Tran, 2009)**.

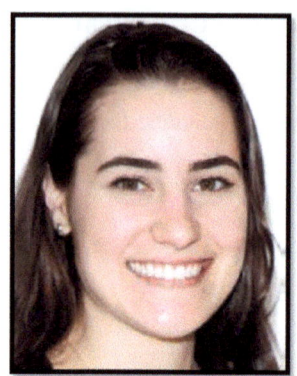

Macro-aesthetics

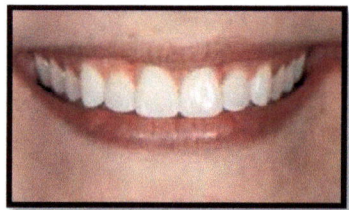
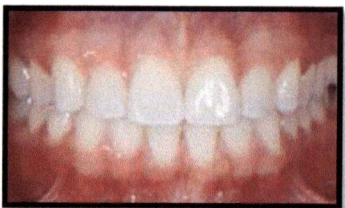

Mini-aesthetics   Micro-aesthetics

Figure 1.6: Classification of Aesthetic Appearance (**Brandão and Brandão, 2013**).

1.1.3. Facial Beauty and Attractiveness

There is an important but proficient difference between facial beauty and facial attractiveness, researchers have agreed that these terms may not always be inter changeable, *Rhee and Koo* in 2007 stated that facial beauty is not a rigid concept, but can evolve and change according to time, generation, age, gender, racial and ethnicity **(Rhee and Koo, 2007)**. On the other hand, facial attractiveness could be objectively measured and defined as the *"time-static visual properties of a face in a photographic two-dimensional frontal repose image that are pleasing to the visual sense of an observer"* **(Bashour, 2006)**.

1.1.3.1. Perceptions of Facial Attractivness

What is perception? Technically, perception is a single, united awareness obtained from sensory processes while the stimulus is present **(Urdang, 1968)**.

Perceptions of an attractive face are questionable, some debate perceptions of attraction were subjective while some debate perceptions of attraction could be measured, subjective believers stated that the personal feelings, culture or combinations of traits that give pleasure to the senses or mind influence perceptions **(Naini *et al.*, 2006)**. Additionally, subjective believers intended that perceptions of attraction reflect individual opinion and could be influenced by society, it has been suggested that minority groups seek to look like majority groups and patients seek to look like fashion models and hollywood celebrities **(Giddon, 1983)**.

There is evidence to suggest that perception of attractivness has a genetic basis, *Rubenstein* found that even at 6 months old infants show a predilection for attractive faces, and because 6 months old is too early in human development for social influences; *Rubenstein* concluded that the reason the infants prefer an attractive face was due to the way our brains were wired, so called "general information processing mechanisms" **(Rubenstein *et al.*, 1999)**

It has been reported that there may be an intrinsic feature common to all beautiful things and that beautiful faces may display a varying amounts of this feature whether it is harmony or balance, so that, researchers have long discussed what constitutes attractiveness **(Iliffe, 1960; Peck and Peck, 1970)**.

Personality, personal appearance, in addition to how an individual behaves, the manner in which they relate to and communicate with others and their ability to make friends was suggested to contribute to an individual's attractiveness, society assesses individuals on these features **(Hilhorst, 2002)**.

Facial attractiveness and expressive behaviour was reported to have the most influence on perception of attractiveness, while body attractiveness and attractiveness of dress had little influence on overall initial judgments of attractiveness **(Riggio *et al.*, 1991)**.

There were different facial features which believed to be assessed subconsciously, when evaluating facial attractiveness and aesthetics.

- Symmetry.
- Youthfulness and neoteny of the face.
- Sexual dimorphism secondary to sex hormones.
- Averageness of facial configurations.

Over the years, symmetry was regarded an important, if not the most important determinant of the facial beauty or attractiveness, a number of studies have supported the idea that the perfect facial symmetry is the cornerstone of facial beauty **(Faure *et al.*, 2002)**; symmetry thought to be a reflection of the quality of one's genes, such that the greater the facial symmetry the greater the ability of one's genes to create a symmetrical individual, an association has been reported between facial symmetry and ratings of attractiveness, more symmetrical faces were appeared to be more attractive and these individuals were considered to be more sociable, balanced, intelligent and self-confident, while those with faces that were less symmetrical were perceived as being more anxious **(Fink *et al.*, 2006).**

Youthfulness was associated with attractiveness and appeared to be more attractive than older faces **(Mathes *et al.*, 1985; Sarwer *et al.*, 2003)**. Whereas, neoteny was associated with babyish features like large eyes, small nose, round cheeks and smooth skin, some studies have shown that neotenous facial features were thought to be more attractive **(Cunningham, 1999).**

There is an evolutionary association between sexual dimorphism (secondary to sex hormones) and facial attractiveness **(Weeden and Sabini, 2005)**. This was assessed further in a study which females asked to rate the attractiveness and symmetry of white and black photographs of forty men's faces, they found two predictors of male attractiveness other than symmetry, namely a prominent cheek bones and longer lower face **(Scheib *et al.*, 1999).**

The idea that averageness was an essential requirement of facial beauty appeared in the early to mid 20th century **(Faure *et al.*, 2002)**. *Langlois* stated that composite images of the face made up of average features were rated as being more attractive than the actual face from which they were created **(Langlois *et al.*, 1994)**. These findings were supported by the concept that the facial attractiveness was associated with facial symmetry and average facial characteristics **(Thornhill and Gangestad, 1999)**. Other researchers found that there were some non-average characteristics that are attractive, and attractiveness is not completely determined by average facial features **(Alley *et al.*, 1991; Perrett *et al.*, 1994; DeBruine *et al.*, 2007)**. The most attractive faces appear to have certain *"distinguishing features"* which transfer upon their owners a particularly high degree of attractiveness **(Jabir, 2014)**.

1.1.3.2. Distinguishing Features

A number of distinguishing features have been suggested, these varied from facial features such as the forehead, cheeks, lips and eyes to dental aesthetics *(well-shaped, correctly inclined or slightly protruding anterior teeth were regarded to be attractive),* there is also a gender specific characteristics, the female face is considered more attractive if it has full lips, thin eyebrows, large eyes, prominent cheek bones, and a small chin and nose **(Faure *et al.*, 2002)**.

In addition to these gender specific characteristics, "a particularly attractive female face would have to incorporate an innocently childlike appearance which appeals to protective instincts but at the same time mature, showing dominance as well as being expressive" **(Swaddle and Cuthill, 1995)**. Men on the other hand were considered to be attractive if they have features such as prominent cheek bones, large jaws, a strong chin, thin lips and thick eyebrows **(Edler, 2001)**. When it comes to male faces, it appears that it is harder to define their attractiveness than in the females as women were affected by a number of other factors such as their menstrual cycle and environment **(Langlois *et al.*, 1987)**.

1.1.3.3. Social Importance of Facial Aesthetics

The face is the most noticeable feature and has a unique influence on how we assess attractiveness in others and how we identify one another **(Riggio et al., 1991)**. Facial appearance is the focus of attention in social interaction , we depend on its information to form first impressions of other people and without further interaction is the basis on how we judge others **(Cunningham, 1999)**, for example, attractive children tend to be perceived more positively by their parents **(Langlois et al., 1995)**, while teachers perceive more attractive children as being more intelligent **(Clifford and Walster, 1973)** and in professional life, less attractive adults are perceived as having fewer qualifications and have less potential for employment success **(Hosoda et al., 2003)**. In addition to that, individuals with Class II malocclusions and mandibular retrognathism may be regarded as weak and possibly idle, whereas those with significant Class III malocclusions and mandibular prognathism may be regarded as aggressive personality types **(Naini et al., 2006)**.

Attractiveness is a visual cue that people use to make hypotheses and conclusions about the personality and behavior of others in once-off encounters and it can influence how we treat other, in modern society, physical beauty is considered as a personal characteristic and is valued as such in its own right, independent of other traits **(Hilhorst, 2002)**.

1.1.4. Soft Tissue of the Face
1.1.4.1. Soft Tissue Changes with Growth

Behrents documented that craniofacial growth did not stop in young adulthood but it is a continuous process that continue into a later ages **(Behrents, 1986)**.

The form of human skeleton is usually beautified by the soft tissue drape **(Premkumar, 2011)**. Whereas the position of the underlying hard tissue is a primary determinant of the overlying soft tissue morphology, this is true for the lips and teeth, chin and bony chin projection, malar prominence and cheeks, growth of the face is a complex function of the skeletal, dental and soft tissue growth; with genetic and environmental factors both playing a significant roles in the final facial form, the most important parts to be discussed are the nose, lips and chin because *"the balance among these three anatomical structures can be altered by both growth and orthodontic treatment"* **(Sarver, 1997).**

1.1.4.2. The Nose

Subtelny-who measured longitudinal soft tissue growth changes of the upper and lower lips, the nose and the soft tissue chin-documented that the downward and forward growth of the nose occurred during maturity, *Subtelny* found that in both genders the vertical dimension of the nose experienced proportionately more growth than the anteroposterior projection **(Subtelny, 1959).**

Generally the girls have tendency to have slightly more nasal growth than boys do during the early period of adolescence, as shown in **(Fig 1.7)**, however, the total incremental increase of nasal growth for boys was greater through ages 10 to 16 years, the majority of growth in length of nasal bone had happened before age 10 years, but the soft tissues have grown downward and forward with maxillary complex **(Manera and Subtelny, 1961; Sarver, 1998).**

The nasal projection in the males from ages 12 to 17 years continued with a greater degree of nasal prominence in males of age 17 years, while the females had completed a large portion of their nasal growth by age 12 years **(Genecov *et al.*, 1990).** The nose is one of the important components of the facial aesthetics, the study of its form is of great importance in plastic surgery **(Costa *et al.*, 2005)** and forensic facial reconstruction **(Stephan *et al.*, 2003; Rodríguez, 2004).**

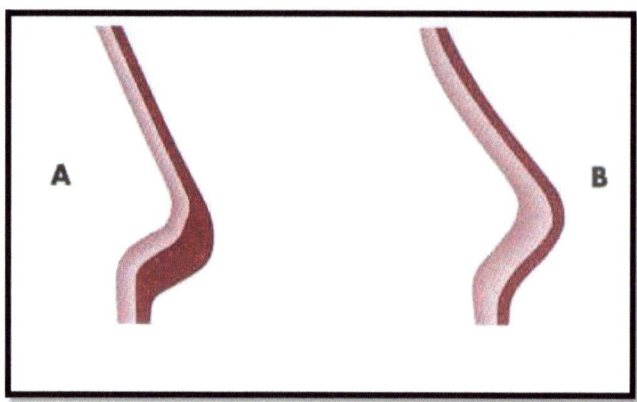

Figure 1.7: Nasal growth, pink coloured area shows growth between 10-13 years of age; red coloured area shows growth between 13-16 years of age. (A) male (B) female.
(Sarver, 1998)

1.1.4.3. The Lips

According to *Subtelny*, the upper lip showed a rapid increase in length from approximately age one to three years, but the rate of incremental growth is significantly reduced between age three and six years **(Subtelny, 1959)**.

The lower anterior facial height (the vertical skeletal and dentoalveolar growth) in adolescents between age 4 and 20 years was concluded before completion of the vertical lip growth; both upper and lower lips grew more than skeletal lower face, the lower lip grew vertically more than upper lip **(Vig and Cohen, 1979)**.

Genecov found that males between ages 7 and 17 years had greater increase in upper lip length than females in same period; the males experienced a little more than 2 mm in vertical height of upper lip and the females experienced less than 1 mm in vertical height of upper lip, while after age 12 years, little vertical lip growth occurred in females between age 12 and 17 years **(Genecov *et al.*, 1990)**.

In both genders, the upper lip usually attained proportionately greater thickness in vermilion region than the region overlying point A, in both male and female from age 1 to 14 years the upper lip was observed to increase in thickness, after the subjects have aged 14 years, the males continued to show an increase in the upper lip thickness, whereas the upper lip did not become discernibly thicker in the females **(Fig 1.8)**, similarly, the increase in lower lip thickness was greater in vermilion region than at Pogonion (Pg) and point B, when subjects were from 1 to 18 years, measurements from the most anterior point of vermilion border of lower lip showed an average increase of 6 mm for females and 7 mm for males **(Subtelny, 1959)**.

According to *Nanda* in 1990, the upper lip thickness increased rather uniformly from age 7-18 years, females experienced the attainment of full lip thickness at age 13 years, with slight thinning beginning at that age, in males, the lip thickness continued on an upward curve until age 18 years **(Nanda et al., 1990)**. *Formby* documented that soft tissue changes in the nose, lips, and chin continued in both males and females even after the age of 25 years **(Formby et al., 1994)**.

1.1.4.4. The Chin

Three factors determind the chin projection, the amount of anteroposterior bony projection of the anterior, inferior border of the mandible and the amount of soft tissue that overlays that bony projection **(Sarver et al., 2000)**.

Nanda in 1955, found that the males exprienced larger incremental changes than females between age 7 and 15 years and the males showed more mandibular growth, which resulted in increased projection of the chin, although the soft tissue thickness of chin itself was roughly parallel, therefore; increased chin projection seen in males during growth was due to more mandibular growth than to soft tissue changes **(Nanda, 1955)**.

Soft tissue chin thickness in females from ages 7 to 9 was 11.7 mm, while in males was 10.8 mm, measured from pogonion (Pg) to soft tissue pogonion (Pg'), **(Fig 1.8)**, but females had only a 1.6 mm increase up to age 17, whereas males had a 2.4 mm increase in tissue thickness over this period, as a result both genders had similar soft tissue chin thickness 13.3 mm at age 17 years **(Genecov *et al.*, 1990; Milošević *et al.*, 2006)**.

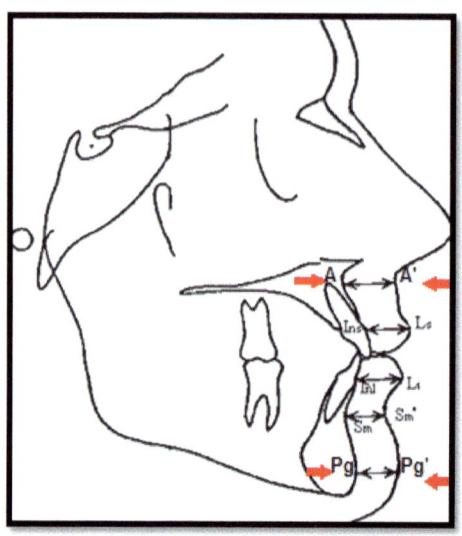

Figure 1.8: Soft tissue landmarks and horizontal variables for measuring the thickness of the upper lip and soft tissue chin, A'-A:Thickness of the upper lip in landmark A' (The landmark of the greatest concavity on the middle upper lip between the subnasale point and labrale superius), Pg'-Pg: Thickness of the soft tissue of the chin in landmark Pg' (Milošević et al., 2006).

1.1.4.5. Height and Width of the Face

Bishara analyzed the growth in height of the facial soft tissues, length of the face continued to increase from childhood to adolescence, the study was conducted for 9 years and the facial length in that period increased by 22.7% in females and 25% in males, the study was made on facial photographs of boys and girls at different ages (4 to 13 years), the assessment was made of the facial profile and frontal view photographs, length and width of the face were assessed, bizygomatic width increased about 9.5% in females and 8.8% in males, intergonial width of the face also increased but the rate of growth slowed after the first year, according to *Ricketts*, "all the facial structures grow in proportion to each other and they follow the divine proportion", **(Premkumar, 2011)**.

1.2. The Dentition
1.2.1. Normal Occlusion

Since the mid of 1920, many concepts of a "perfect" or "ideal" occlusion had been suggested **(Friel, 1927; Ramfjord and Ash, 1966; Stuart, 1967; Huffman et al., 1969; Andrews, 1972)**. An ideal occlusion is a theoretical or hypothetical concept that based on anatomy of the teeth and in nature it is rarely found, the ideal occlusion concept was applied to a condition when the maxilla and mandible skeletal bases were in correct size relative to each other and the teeth should be in a correct relationship in all three planes of space at rest, it could be precisely described and could be used as a standard by which other occlusions types could be judged **(McDonald & Ireland, 1998; Nanda, 2015)** as shown in **(Fig 1.9)**.

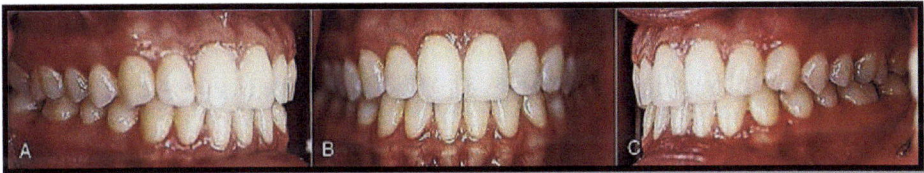

Figure 1.9: Frontal and lateral views of an ideal occlusion: A- right side, B- ftontal, C- left side **(Nanda, 2015)**.

Edward Angle in the 1890, was the first who defined the normal occlusion; which is based on the mesiobuccal cusp of the maxillary first permanent molar **(Moyers, 1988; Proffit et al., 2007)**, **(Fig 1.10)**. *Houston* in 1992 defined the normal occlusion as an occlusion within an accepted deviation of the ideal and did not constitute aesthetic or functional problems **(Houston et al., 1992)**.

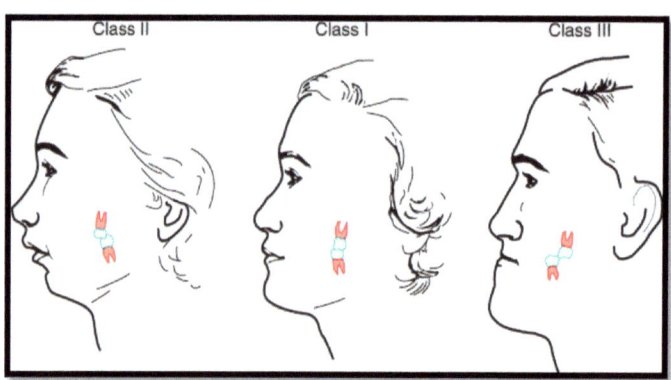

Figure 1.10: Angle classification, Facial profile and molar relationship **(Moyers, 1988)**.

For a normal occlusion to exist, the size of the teeth must be normal, tooth size is defined by the width and length of a particular tooth, the width is the largest mesiodistal distance perpendicular to the long axis of the tooth, while the length is the largest distance along the long axis of the tooth from the incisal edge to the gingival margin, the size of the teeth was often expressed as the relationship between the width and the length, known as the width/length ratio, there were a marked range of tooth sizes in a population **(Rose, 2013)**. *Magne* in 2003 found that the maxillary central incisor average width was to be 9.1 mm with a range of 8.4 mm to 11.1 mm **(Magne *et al.*, 2003)**, whereas *Gillen* in 1994 found that the average length of maxillary central incisor was to be 10.4 mm **(Gillen *et al.*, 1994)**.

Wayne Bolton **(Bolton, 1962)**, was the first one who described the "tooth-size analysis ratios" which could be defined by "the relative size of the teeth compared to each other", *Bolton* found that the sum of the sizes of the mandibular anterior teeth were related to the sum of the sizes of maxillary anterior teeth by the following ratio:

$$\text{Anterior Ratio} = \frac{\text{Sum of mandibular anterior teeth}}{\text{Sum of maxillary anterior teeth}} * 100$$

CHAPTER ONE — Review of Literature

The anterior ratio equaled to 77.6% in untreated cases with excellent occlusion, the mandibular anterior teeth were larger or the maxillary anterior teeth were smaller when this ratio is higher than normal, this may lead to a reduction in overjet and overbite, creating an open bite or end to end incisor occlusion, if the anterior ratio is smaller than normal, then either the maxillary teeth were larger or mandibular teeth were smaller, smaller than average ratio lead to increased overjet and overbite **(Bolton, 1962; Sarver and Yanosky, 2005)**.

1.2.2. Dental Aesthetics

Although the field of dental aesthetics is a complicated branch and may be regarded to be purely subjective; this 'subjective' branch of dentistry encompassed by rules and values that allow us to study it objectively, however "perception of dental aesthetics varies from person to person and is influenced by their personal experience and social environment" **(Rosenstiel, 2000)**, this statement was further backed up by the findings of *Hunt* in 2002, who stated that people who attend the dentist regularly have higher dental aesthetic ambitions **(Hunt *et al.*, 2002)**.

It is important to start at the beginning, when man first studied the art of beauty, in the period 365-300BC, the Egyptians and the Greeks started to understand the divine or golden proportion that known as *a golden ratio* "which is the ratio of 1: 1.618 that considered to be the most aesthetically pleasing to the human eye and the base of countless mysteries over centuries" to design their great pyramids and parthenon respectively **(Peck and peck, 1970; Matoulla and Panshez, 2006; Mahadevia *et al.*, 2010)**.

Lombardi stated that the repeated ratio means that the existing proportion between the width of the central incisor and lateral incisor should be constant, progressing anteriorly to posteriorly **(Lombardi, 1973)**.

Levin was one of the first people who applied the golden proportion to the smile, documented that the mesiodistal width of maxillary lateral incisor should be in a golden proportion to the mesiodistal width of the maxillary central incisor, the lateral incisor should be 62% of the width of the maxillary central incisor, and the maxillary canine should be 62% of the width of the maxillary lateral incisor **(Levin, 1978; Proffit *et al.*, 2013)** as shown in **(Fig 1.11)**.

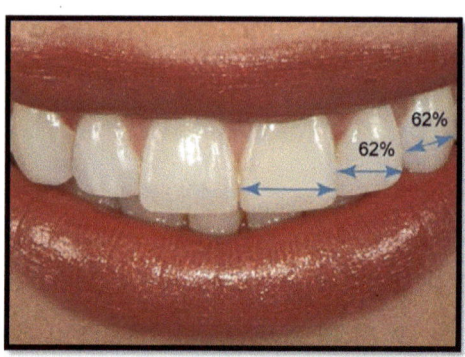

Figure 1.11: Ideal tooth width proportions when viewed from the front (Proffit et al., 2013).

Recently, *Ward* showed in his survey that the recurring esthetic dental (RED) proportion means the proportion of successive widths of the maxillary anterior teeth should remain constant as viewed from the front, progressing distally, this proportion did not have a fixed value **(Ward, 2008)**. *Ward* reported that 57% of the dentists surveyed preferred smiles with the 70% recurring esthetic dental (RED) proportion and according to *Ward*, when using the 70% RED proportion, the mesiodistal width of the maxillary lateral incisor is 70% of the frontal view of the maxillary central incisor, and the maxillary canine is 70% of the width of the maxillary lateral incisor, the preferred width-to-height ratio determined in his study was 78%, with an acceptable range of 60% to 80% **(Ward, 2007)**.

Preston in 1993 **(Preston, 1993)**, studied the presence of golden proportion in natural dentition and documented that only 17% of maxillary lateral incisors width were in a golden proportion with the width of the maxillary central incisors and none of canines width were in a golden proportion to the width of the maxillary lateral incisor, so Preston's proportion exist when the width of maxillary lateral incisor is 66% of the width of maxillary central incisors and the width of maxillary canine is 55% of the width of the maxillary central incisors in the frontal view **(Mahshid et al., 2004; Shetty et al., 2011)** as shown in **(Fig 1.12)**.

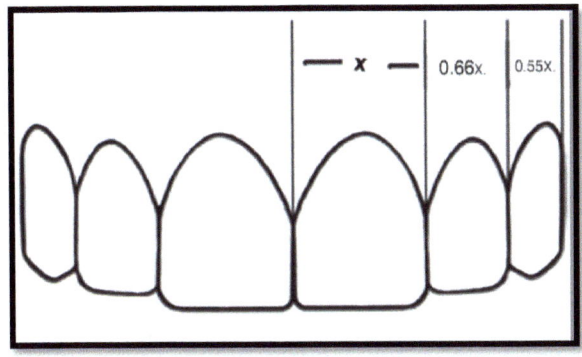

Figure 1.12: Preston's proportion: Calculating the width of the maxillary anterior teeth using Preston's proportion, "X" represent the mesiodistal width of maxillary central incisor **(Shetty et al., 2011)**.

According to *Gillen*, these values hold true regardless of race and gender **(Gillen et al., 1994)**, whereas *Touati* suggested that each anterior maxillary tooth plays a specific aesthetic role that central incisors provide stability and balance, lateral incisors provide charm, and canines bring strength into the aesthetic zone **(Touati, 1998)**.

1.2.2.1. Dental Aesthetics and Maxillary Anterior Teeth

Dental aesthetics is considered an important part of successful dental treatment, especially in treatment involving a patient's smile **(Konikoff and Johnson, 2007)**. The maxillary central incisor is considered the most important tooth due to it's prominent position in the front of the dentition, the ideal aesthetics of the maxillary central incisors have been studied in terms of position, size, and relationship to other teeth **(Sarver, 2004; Hasanreisoglu et al, 2005)**.

Some studies have identified limits for what is considered aesthetic, according to *Kokich*, the central incisor was considered by laypeople to be unaesthetic when it is 2.0 mm shorter than its ideal length **(Kokich *et al*, 1999)**. The width/length ratio of the central incisor is most attractive between 75-85% **(Wolfart *et al*., 2005; Cooper *et al*., 2012)**, while according to *Sarver* and *Gurel* the ideal maxillary central incisor width should be approximately 80% compared with height **(Gurel, 2003; Sarver, 2004), (Fig 1.13)**, but it has been reported to vary between 66% and 80% **(Gillen *et al*., 1994)**.

A higher width/height ratio means a squarer tooth, and a lower ratio means a longer appearance, although the range of height and width is important to note; these measurements should not be taken as an absolute rule as many smiles shows disproportionality **(Shillingburg *et al*., 1972; Mavroskoufis and Ritchie, 1980)**. Because of the disproportionality of a tooth could be evaluated with regard to what parameter was at fault and in need of improvement; extensive changes in tooth proportions were needed when one tooth is to substitute for another and the most frequent is the substitution of maxillary canine for congenitally missing lateral Incisor **(Katti *et al*., 2013)**.

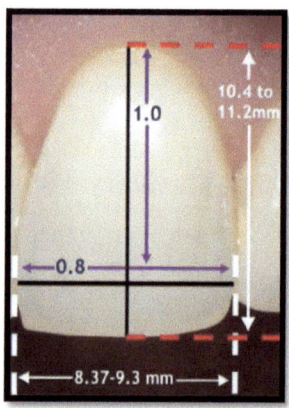

Figure 1.13: Height-width proportions for maxillary central incisors, with normal range of width and height, the width of the tooth should be about 80% of it's height (Sarver, 2004).

The position of the teeth is another aesthetic consideration, a majority of beautiful smiles show 75-100% of the central incisor crown **(Al-Johany et al., 2011)**. The ideal proportions of the teeth to each other is a topic of debate, the divine "golden" proportion in dental aesthetics is based on the Fibonacci sequence: 0, 1, 1, 2, 3, 5, 8, 13, 21, 34, 55, 89, 144, 233, 377…to infinity, these numbers were known as Fibonacci numbers and each new number in this sequence is the sum of the previous two numbers in a way that the farther the number sequence goes, the closer it gets to the golden proportion. **(Ricketts, 1982c; Nikgoo et al., 2009, Saraf and Saraf, 2013).**

Snow considered a bilateral analysis of the apparent individual tooth width as a percentage of a total apparent width of the six maxillary anterior teeth, the *"golden percentage"* suggests that the mesiodistal width of the maxillary central incisor is 25% of the perceived intercanine distance, the perceived width of the lateral incisors is 15% and the canines is 10% **(Snow, 1999; Calçada et al., 2014)**, as shown in **(Fig 1.14)**.

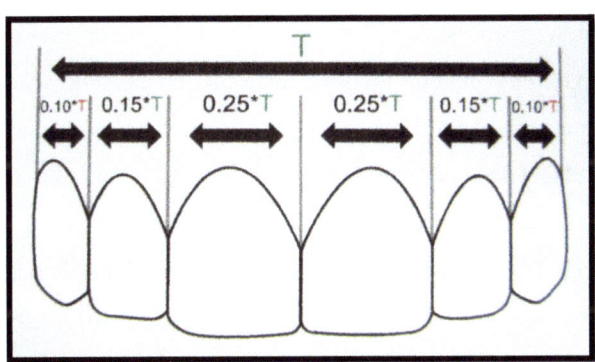

Figure 1.14: Golden percentage, (T) represents the intercanine distance (Calçada et al., 2014)

The contact between the maxillary anterior teeth is done in a descending fashion, beginning from the maxillary canine, the contact between the maxillay canine and the lateral incisor was positioned higher than the contact between the maxillary lateral and the central incisors; the contact between the maxillary central incisors is even lower **(Câmara, 2010)**. The contact points should be narrow, unless there were a discrepancy in the mesiodistal diameter of the crown **(Andrews, 1989)**. Additionally, the golden ratio was applied to the height of contact points of the anterior teeth **(Morley and Eubank, 2001; Sarver, 2004; Sarver, 2011)**. The position of the contact points between the maxillary anterior teeth is related to the tooth position and form **(Magne *et al.*, 2003)**.

The location where the anterior teeth appear to touch is known as a connecting space, there is a difference between the *connecting space* and the *contact point*, the *contact points* were small areas in which teeth actually touch **(Sarver, 2004)**, whereas *connecting spaces* were broader, larger, and could be defined as a zones in which the two adjacent teeth were appeared to touch, according to *Morley and Eubank*, the best aesthetic relationship for the connecting space of the maxillary anterior teeth should follow the 50-40-30 rule, so that the connecting space between the maxillary central incisors should be 50% of the height of those teeth, the ideal connecting space between the maxillary central and the lateral incisor is 40% of the height of the maxillary central incisors, and the connecting space between the maxillary canine and the lateral incisor is 30% of the same reference **(Morley and Eubank, 2001), (Fig 1.15)**.

Although the reference points to determine the connecting space were not well defined by *Morley and Eubank*; these references could be formed by the contact points line and the papillary line which is formed by the tips of gingival papillae that located between the maxillary canines and the lateral incisors, and between the maxillary lateral incisors and the central incisors **(Kurth and Kokich, 2001; Tarnow *et al.*, 1992)**. When using the papillary line and the contact points line as a reference, a band named as *"connector band"* will be obtained, it is called so because the figure of this band resembles a shape of a "hang glider", small changes in this band could make a difference in the dental aesthetics **(Câmara, 2010)** as shown in **(Fig 1.16)**.

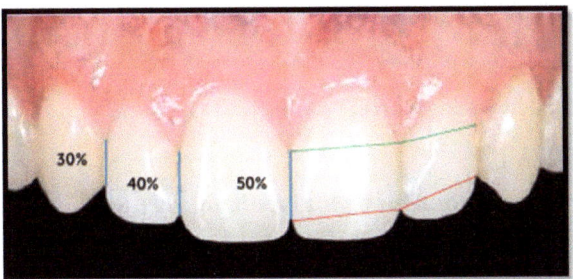

Figure 1.15: Ideal heights of contact points, it must be half of the height of the crown of the central incisors and decreasing distally **(Câmara, 2010)**.

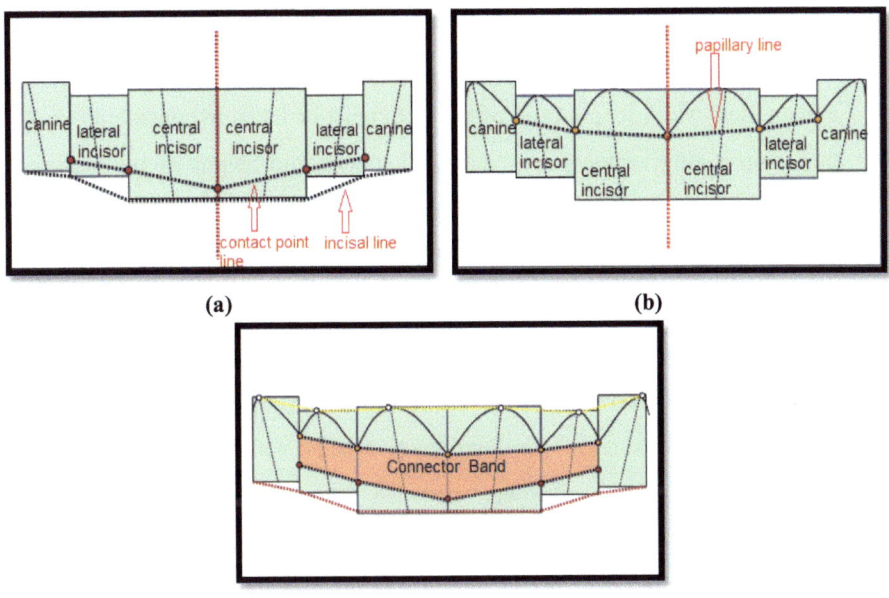

Figure 1.16: Height of the contact points, (a) contact points line should be parallel to the incisal line, (b) papillary line consists of the tips of gingival papillae, (c) connector band is determined by the contact points line and papillary line and it is resembles the shape of a "hang glider" **(Câmara, 2010)**.

According to *Kina and Bruguera* **(Kina and Bruguera, 2007)**, the hypothetical line that connect the ends of the anterior contact points must be parallel to the horizontal lines of the face and to the edge of the lower lip in order to establish a harmonious and cohesive unity of the smile. The most important connector area is the one between two maxillary central incisors and should be maintained in orthodontically treated cases **(Katti *et al*., 2013)**.

There were three ways to achieve the aesthetic relationship for the connecting space of the anterior teeth:

- ✓ **Prosthetic increase:** is selective for the crowns height of the anterior teeth, the procedures of restorative dentistry, specially the porcelain veneers were increasingly used and resistant to time **(Kina *et al*., 2007; Adolfi, 2009)**.
- ✓ **Gingivectomy including the papilla**: the correction of the gingival contour and an ideal width/length ratio of the teeth must be taken in consideration when performing gingivectomy by "intervening with the height of the interdental papilla", but it is important to avoid the opening of the black spaces in the interdental spaces **(Tarnow *et al*., 1992)**.
- ✓ **Ameloplasty:** performed in two ways, either by increasing the contact area by interdental reduction, or reducing the contact area of incisal edges that lead to alter the incisal spaces **(Sarver, 2011)**. According to *Magne and Belser*, the interdental embrasures form interdental angles which were shaped as an inverted "V" shape, narrower between the maxillary central incisors, asymmetric between the maxillary central and the lateral and larger between the maxillary lateral incisor and canine **(Magne and Belser, 2001)**.

1.2.3. Dentofacial Relationships

Knowledge of dentofacial relationships aids in the selection of important dental characteristics, such as central incisor width and intercanine width, so in dentistry, it is important to establish a relationship between the size of the teeth and the rest of the face, inspite of the number of dentofacial relationships and the evidence supporting them, there is still a variability in the size of the teeth so that the relationships were not always accurate **(Mavroskoufis and Ritchie, 1980; Zlataric et al., 2007)**.

Bizygomatic width is one of the horizontal facial dimensions that used in dentofacial relationships **(Fig 1.17:1)**, the distance between points located on the right and left zygomas is 16 times the mesiodistal width of the maxillary central incisor **(Gomes et al., 2006; Ellakwa et al., 2011; Kumar et al., 2011; Proffit et al., 2013)**, and of 1:3.3 of the maxillary anterior teeth width **(Zarb et al., 1990)**. Whereas the facial height which is the vertical distance from nasion to menton has a 1:11 ratio to the length of the maxillary central incisor **(Kern, 1967; Lavere et al., 1992)**.

A second horizontal facial dimension is the interpupillary distance **(Fig 1.17:4)**, the distance between the center of the right and left pupils is reported to be 6.6 times the mesiodistal width of the maxillary central incisor **(Wehner et al., 1967; Verma et al., 1978; Cesario and Latta, 1984; Gomes et al., 2006; Proffit et al., 2013)**. *Cesario and Latta* in their study suggested and evaluated the *interpupillary distance* and the mesiodistal width of the maxillary central incisor, they divided the subjects into four categories: white male and female, and black male and female, *Cesario and Latta* found that the ratio of 1:6.6 fall within the 95% of three of the four groups, while the fourth (black male) the ratio was reported to be 1:7 **(Cesario and Latta, 1984)**. Whereas the Intercanthal which is the distance between the right and left medial canthus, is in a golden proportion to the width of the two maxillary central incisors **(Kumar et al., 2011)**. The intercanthal distance could be related to 4 mesiodistal width combinations of the maxillary anterior teeth **(Al Wazzan, 2001; Proffit et al., 2013)**, **(Fig 1.17:3)**.

The intercanine distance which is the distance measured from cusp tip to cusp tip may be predicted by using the interalar distance **(Hasanreisoglu et al., 2005; Gomes et al., 2006; Gomes et al., 2009; Ellakwa et al., 2011)**, that is measured between the outer points of the ala of the nose in a straight line, corresponding to the morphological width of the nose **(Leong and White 2004; Leong and White, 2006)**.

Mouth width is the distance between the two angles of the mouth (mouth commissure), from chilion to chilion (**Proffit *et al.*, 2013**), **(Fig 1.17:6)**, *Silverman* **(Silverman, 1967)** indicated that the distal surface of maxillary canines were 4 mm away from mouth commissures. This method is based on the hypothesis that the distal surface of the maxillary canines should be approximately located at the corners of the mouth **(Zarb *et al.*, 1990)**.

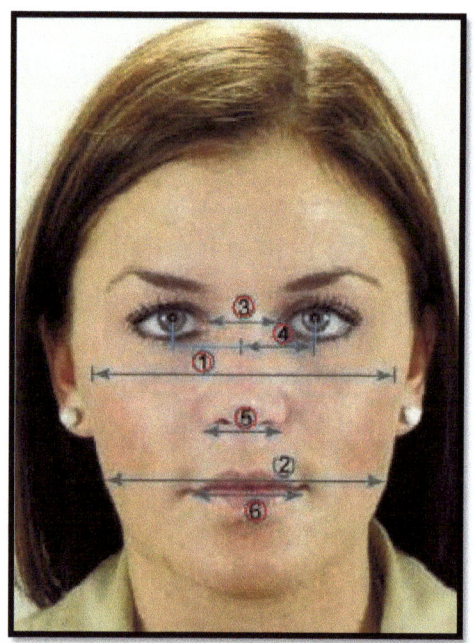

Figure 1.17: Horizontal facial dimension, 1: zygomatic width, 2: gonial width, 3: intercanthal distance, 4: interpupillary width, 5: interalar width, 6: mouth width **(Proffit *et al.*, 2013).**

1.3. Methods of Facial Measurements

Various methods of facial analysis result in many linear and angular measurements, the absolute values of facial measurements were not as important as proportionality **(Reynecke and Ferretti, 2012)**, the most important methods of facial measurements are:

1.3.1. Direct methods

1.3.1.a. Craniometry

Physical measurement of dry skulls *"Craniometry"*, and sometimes known as craniology was one of the first scientific methods for deriving measurements of the head and neck, this method was used by ancient Greek, but the use of measurements to compare skulls was not developed until the 17th century **(Findlay, 1980)**.

The modern and quantitative study of craniometry was obtained essentially from the 19th century, when it became widely accepted that the theories of evolution could be explored through detailed comparisons of the skulls, but with craniometry, measurements from an individual skull that represent a single time-point and longitudinal data that evaluating changes during growth were not possible **(premkumar, 2011; Payne, 2013), (Fig 1.18)**.

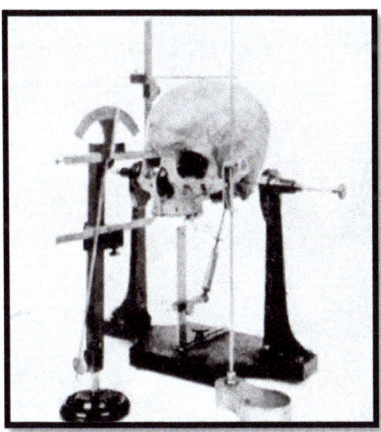

Figure 1.18: Apparatus used for craniometry devised in 1902 **(premkumar, 2011)**.

1.3.1.b. Anthropometry

Anthropometry has been developed when craniometry showed inability to measure longitudinal changes, anthropometry was obtained from the Greek words "anthropos" meaning human and "metron" meaning "to measure"; and it is the biologic science used in measuring size, weight, and proportions of the body **(Farkas, 1998)**. *Hrdlicka* was considered the "father of medical anthropology", he used calipers and rulers to record direct facial measurements from individuals over an extended period of time **(Hrdlicka, 1920)**.

Furthermore, anthropometric standards were developed by *Farkas*, by taking measurements of individuals of various ethnicities in addition to 2500 Caucasian Canadians **(Farkas 1994; Farkas *et al.*, 2005)**.

The use of anthropometric measurements in orthodontics was also adopted in the early 20th century which provided a standardized and comprehensive method to evaluate facial aesthetics and quantify changes to facial structures during growth and treatment **(Hellman, 1939)**.

Anthropometric measurements were still being used to quantitatively measure different aspects of aesthetics in orthodontics, such as dimensions of the teeth and characteristics of the smile but indirect techniques have been used more frequently in the orthodontic field **(Sarver, 2004; Proffit *et al.*, 2013), (Fig 1.19)**.

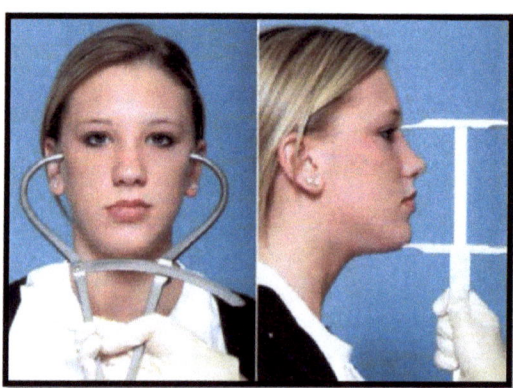

Figure 1.19: Anthropometric analysis for facial measurements **(Proffit *et al.*, 2013)**.

1.3.2. Indirect methods
1.3.2.a. Cephalometric Analysis

Cephalometric radiographs was introduced by *Broadbent* (**Broadbent 1931**). Cephalometric radiographs, as craniometry, allowed for dentoskeletal structures measurement without interferences from soft tissues of varying thickness (**Park, 1986**).

Bjork documented that additional soft tissue measurements were made with the use of radiographic markers placed on the skin prior to exposing the radiograph (**Bjork, 1955**).

Although the cephalometric radiographs played a major and important role in quantitative diagnosis and treatment planning in orthodontics, and the use of cephalometry offored the ability to measure the soft tissue profile outline and quantify changes over extended period of time from growth and treatment (**Burstone, 1959**); the use of cephalometric radiographs for extended evaluation has limitations, such as cephalometric radiographs were a two-dimensional representation of three-dimensional craniofacial structures, which lead to distortion of dentoskeletal structures based on the plane in which they lie (**Baumrind and Frantz, 1971**) and exposure of patients to ionizing radiation repeatedly has proven to have detrimental and harmful effects, especially when taking progressive radiographs (**Mupparapu, 2005; Fazel *et al.*, 2009; Claus *et al.*, 2012**).

1.3.2.b. Photographical Analysis

Photogrammetry has been used in orthodontics to evaluate the facial proportions and assess changes during orthodontic treatment, photogrammetry means the evaluation of an object by using of a photograph, it is an inexpensive and non-invasive method of quantifying and evaluating facial aesthetics (**Stoner, 1955; Neger, 1959**).

| CHAPTER ONE | Review of Literature |

A series of facial photographs has been a standard part of orthodontic diagnostic records for many years **(Proffit *et al.*, 2013)**. Advances and development in digital photography and computer software have enhanced the usefulness of photographs for quantitative linear and angular facial analysis, photographs could be easily taken from multiple angles, allow facial soft tissue dimensions to be fully assessed and evaluated, this benefit is not possible with cephalometry, digital photographs may be viewed immediately, without waiting for the film negatives to be developed, as well as modified and measured using specialized computer programs **(Payne, 2013)**.

I. **Photographical Technique:** A photographical technique that ensures the best reliable images has to be utilized, and includes:

✓ *Positioning of the head*: Some authors use the Frankfort-Horizontal line "which is considered one of the most appreciable reference line" as a base to position the head **(Leivesley, 1983; Meredith, 1997)**. Others use the natural head position method **(Cooke and Stephen, 1988; Claman *et al.*, 1990; Ferrario *et al.*, 1993; Fernández-Riveiro *et al.*, 2002; Malkoç *et al.*, 2009)**.

✓ *Object-lens distance*: It was found that a distance of 7 feet (about 2.13m) is the most appropriate camera-to-object distance for the photograph to be with least distortion **(Benson and Richmond, 1997)**, while *Meneghini (***Meneghini, 2005)** suggested the (101 cm) as a good distance to give high quality photograph.

✓ *Background*: The appearance of a photographed subject could be changed by the color intensity or cluttering of the background, variation in background could darken shadows or eliminate certain margins of the photographed subject **(Dickason and Hanna, 1976)**. The color of the background varied between investigators, *Dickason and Hanna* found that the most acceptable colors for the background were light blue and gray blue **(Dickason and Hanna, 1976)**.

Morello and Meredith used a light blue green paper **(Morello *et al.*, 1977; Meredith, 1997)**, whereas *Gordon and Wander* considered the light gray or blue as ideal **(Gordon and Wander, 1987)**. Although it is a matter of personal preference, but light shades of colors in general were preferred to get the best contrast **(Howells and Shaw, 1985)**.

II. **Types of photographs used in orthodontics:**
   a. **Facial photographs (extra-oral):** *Graber and Vanarsdall* stated the ideal photographical representation of the face, the following facial photographs were recommended as the expected routine for each patient: **(Graber and Vanarsdall, 2000; Meneghini and Biondi, 2012)** as shown in **(Fig 1.20):**
   - **Frontal view:** This recommended for facial analysis **(Fig 1.20a)**.
   - **Frontal dynamic (smile) view**: This recommended to demonstrate the amount of incisor show on smile (percentage of maxillary incisor display on smile), as well as any excessive gingival display **(Fig 1.20b)**.
   - **Profile view:** This recommended for profile analysis, common method used for positioning the patient properly is to have the patient look in a mirror, orienting the head on the visual axis **(Fig 1.20c)**.
   - **A three-quarter view (45-degree) photograph**: This could be quite useful for examination of the mid-face and is particularly informative of mid-face deformities, including nasal deformity **(Fig 1.20d)**.
   - **A close-up image of the posed smile view:** This is now recommended as a standard photograph for careful analysis of the smile relationships **(Fig 1.20e)**.
   - **An optional submental view:** Such a view may be taken to document mandibular asymmetries **(Fig 1.20f)**.

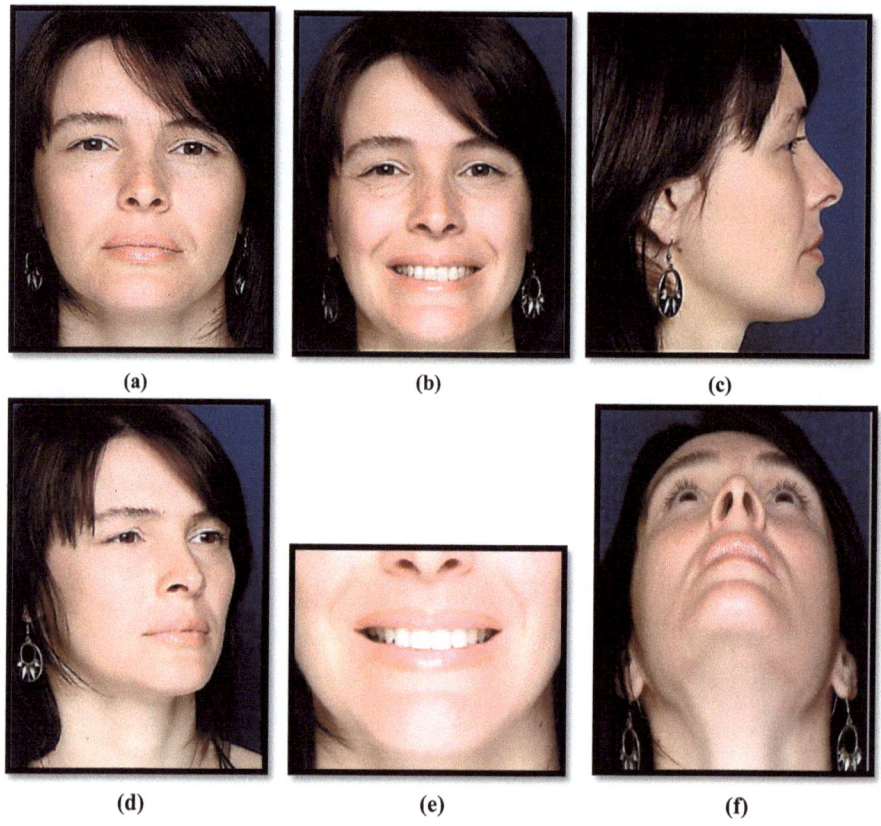

Figure 1.20: Facial photograph (Meneghini and Biondi, 2012).

b. **Intra-oral photographs:** The intra-oral photographical series consists of five views: *right and left lateral* **(Fig 1.21, a, b)**, *frontal* **(Fig 1.21, c)** and *upper and lower occlusal* views **(Fig 1.21, d, e)**, the major purpose of the intra-oral photograph is to enable the orthodontist to review the hard and soft tissue findings at the clinical examination as all the diagnostic data were being analyzed **(Graber and Vanarsdall, 2000; Sandler and Murray, 2002; Graber, 2012).**

| CHAPTER ONE | Review of Literature |

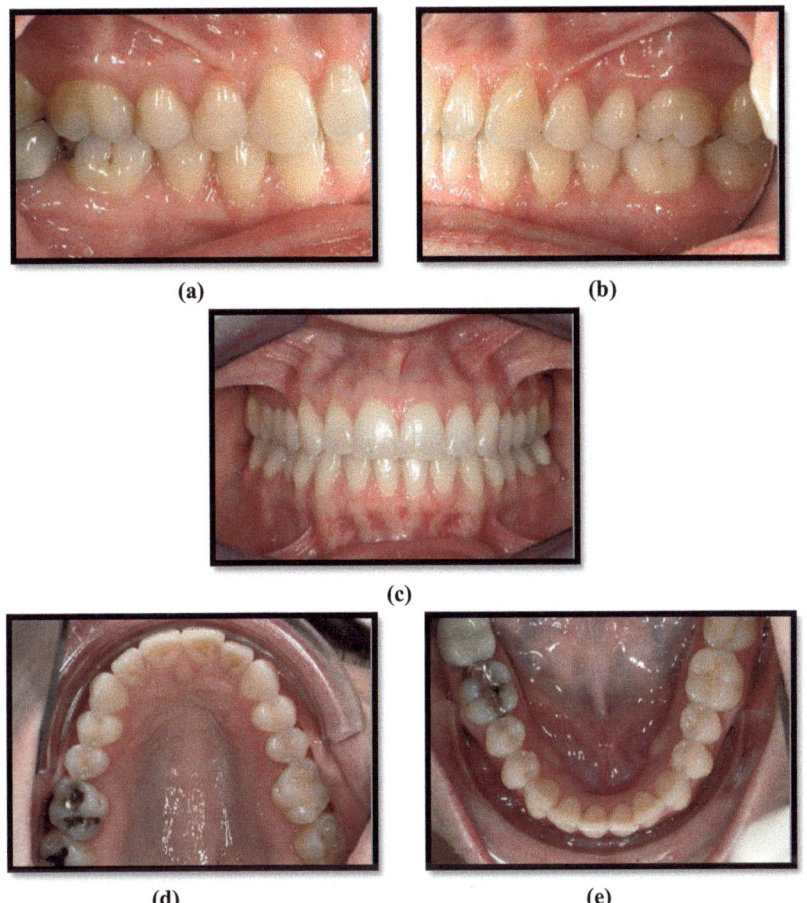

Figure 1.21: Intra-oral photographs, (a): right lateral, (b): left lateral, (c): frontal, (d): upper occlusal, (e): lower occlusal **(Graber, 2012)**.

1.3.2.c. Three-Dimensional Imaging Analysis

Thalmann-Degan in 1944 as cited by **Burke and Beard (1967)**, described the use of *"three-dimensional imaging"* for facial evaluation in orthodontics, three-dimensional imaging offers the three-dimensional benefit of craniometry and anthropometry with the benefit of indirect facial measurement. *Stereophoto-grammetry* is the first technique that used a multiple photogrammetric angles converging on the face, captured together with multiple cameras, to construct the three-dimensional soft-tissue outline **(Hajeer *et al.*, 2004; Karatas, 2014)** as shown in **(Fig 1.22).**

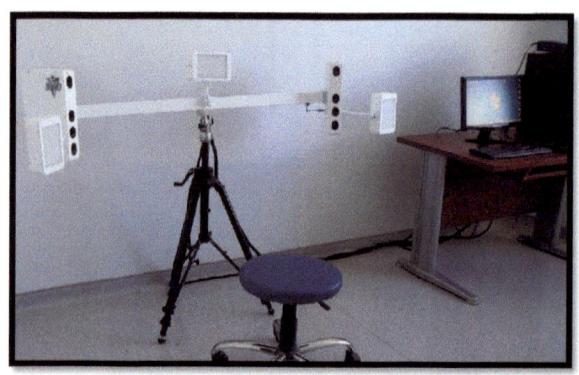

Figure 1.22: Stereophotogrammetry with two different coplanar planes for 3D images (Karatas, 2014).

1.3.2.d. Cone-Beam Computer Tomography Analysis

A scanning laser records facial soft tissue envelope and provide a computerized reconstruction of the face on which measurements could be done, *cone-beam computer tomography (CBCT)* is another three-dimensional technique used for facial soft tissue measurements in orthodontics, CBCT is like craniometry, offors measurements of the dentoskeletal structures of the head, but with the convenience of indirect measurement and measurements of the same individual at different time-points, patients exposure to radiation and minimally visualized facial soft tissue limited CBCT usefulness for evaluation of total facial aesthetics **(Chang *et al.*, 2011).**

1.3.2.e. Video-Imaging Analysis

Video-imaging has been recently used to make a dynamic measurements of facial soft tissues, rather than static measurements from other indirect methods, the video-imaging in orthodontics has been used for measuring dynamic movements of the soft tissue during smile animation, this technique improved visualization of the soft tissue contour by recording the face from different angles **(Sarver, 1996; Sarver and Ackerman, 2003a; Sarver and Ackerman, 2003b).**

1.4. Previous Studies Related to photographical analysis of the facial and dental measurements in Baghdad

- *Al-Ramahi S, Al-Mulla A* in 2009, evaluated the buccal corridor in posed smile for Iraqi adults sample with class I normal occlusion by using photographs.
- *Al-Maliki H, Ali F* in 2011, studied the dental arches dimensions, forms and the relation of dental arch to facial types in a sample of Iraqi adults with skeletal and dental class I normal occlusion by using photographs and dental casts.
- *Hassan D, Ghaib N* in 2011, studied the reliability of bisecting interpupillary perpendicular line, facial and dental laterality and coincidence in Iraqi adults sample with normal occlusion by using photographs and dental casts.
- *Al-Janabi S, Ali F* in 2011, analysed the facial soft tissue profile of Iraqi Adults with Class I normal occlusion by using photographs.
- *Abdulkareem S, Al-Mothaffar N* in 2011, evaluated the accuracy and precision of a photographic system for the three-dimensional study of facial morphology.
- *Ahmed H, Al-Labban Y, Nahidh M* in 2013, by using photograph, they found out the relationship between facial and actual mesiodistal dimensions of maxillary anterior teeth obtained from dental casts.

Chapter Two
Materials and Methods

2.1. Materials
2.1.1. Sample

The sample of this study was achieved from undergraduate students at College of Dentistry-University of Baghdad. After the research purpose was explained to the students and an agreement was obtained from them to participate in this study, they were examined clinically, and out of 450 students examined, only 120 of them (60 females and 60 males) fitted the criteria of sample selection. The sample consisted of 240 frontal photographs (120 extraoral photographs and 120 intraoral photographs).

2.1.1.1. Criteria for Sample Selection

a. Inclusion criteria:
- ✓ All are Iraqies with an age ranged between 18-23 years.
- ✓ All have full permanent dentition regardless the third molars **(Sweirgenga et al., 1994)**.
- ✓ Normal overjet and overbite (2-4 mm), **(Kim et al., 2005)**.
- ✓ Bilateral Class I buccal segments "molar and canine" **(Angle, 1899)**.
- ✓ Skeletal Class I relationship determined clinically by two finger method **(Foster, 1985; Mitchle, 2013)**.
- ✓ No spacing or crowding in the anterior teeth **(Al-Marzok et al., 2013)**.

b. Exclusion criteria:

- ✓ History of facial trauma, orthodontic/orthognathic treatment, dentofacial deformities, surgeries or asymmetry **(Mahmoud, 2010)**.
- ✓ Presence of anterior or posterior crossbite **(Gomes *et al.*, 2009)**.
- ✓ Presence of dental midline shift.
- ✓ Presence of active periodontal diseases and gingivitis **(Abdulhadi and Mohammed, 2012)**.
- ✓ History of bad oral habits like thumb sucking, tongue thrust or mouth breathing **(Al-Zubaydi, 2005)**.
- ✓ Presence of intruded, extruded or rotated teeth in the anterior region **(Parnia *et al.*, 2010)**.
- ✓ Presence of signs of attrition and restoration of the maxillary anterior teeth **(Naqash and Bali, 2013)**.
- ✓ Presence of proximal caries, developmental anomalies such as supernumerary teeth, prosthesis in the anterior teeth **(Jafari *et al.*, 2014)**.

2.1.2. Instruments and Equipments

- Disposable dental mirrors, cotton, gloves, masks, disinfectant (Desident Cavicide, Spofadental), cheek retractor (Orthotechnology, USA) **(Fig 2.1)**.
- Dental vernier (Dentaurum, Germany), pencil, blue marker pen, disposable plastic barriers for ear rods **(Fig 2.1)**.
- Measuring tape to measure the distance between the participants and the camera lens.
- A digital camera (Canon EOS 60D, 18.0 Megapixels, Japan) with (18-200) lens and height adjustable tripod **(Fig 2.2, 2.3)**.
- Two rulers, one for the extraoral photograph and the other one for the intraoral photograph **(Fig 2.4, 2.5)**
- Cephalostat provided with the Planmeca X-ray machine **(Fig 2.6)**.

CHAPTER TWO   Materials and Methods

- Blue background made of a piece of cloth **(Fig 2.6)**.
- Stool **(Fig 2.6)**.
- Dry heat oven (memmert, KG)**.**
- Personal Computer (HP Pavilion tx 2000).
- Analyzing software (AutoCAD, 2014).

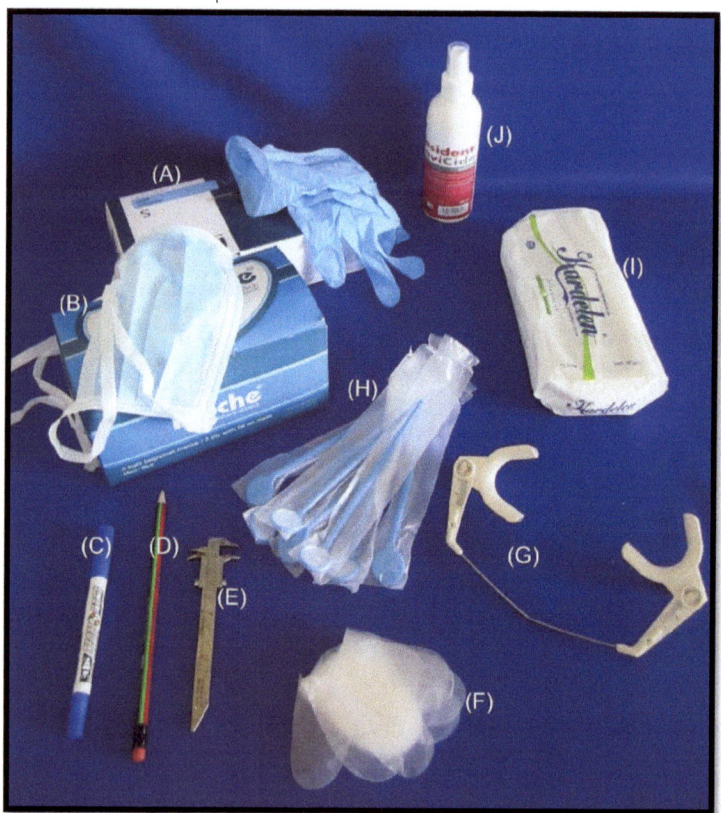

Figure 2.3: Instruments used in the study, (A): Gloves, (B): Masks, (C): Blue Marker Pen, (D): Pencil, (E): Dental Vernier, (F): Disposable Plastic Barriers, (G): Cheek Retractor, (H): Disposable Mirrors, (I): Cotton, (J): Disinfectant.

CHAPTER TWO

Materials and Methods

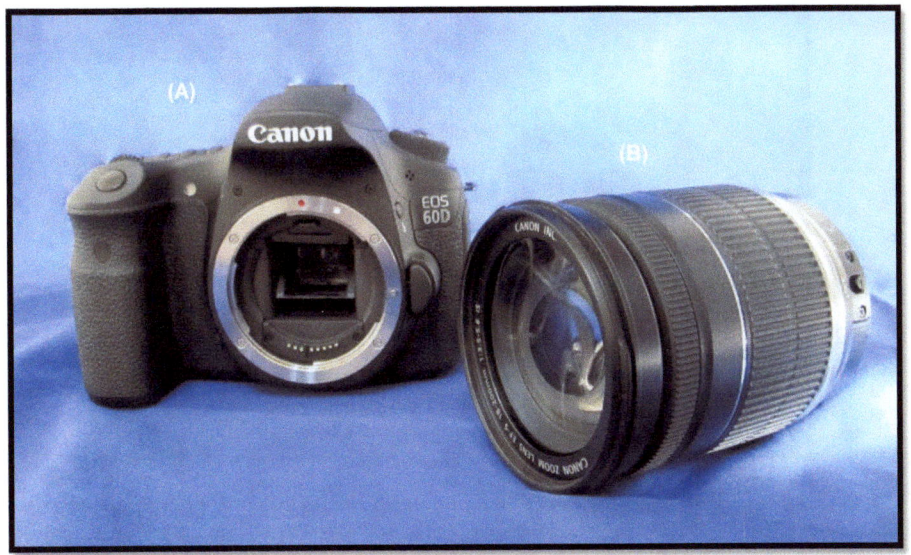

Figure 2.2: (A): A digital camera (Canon EOS 60D), (B): (18-200) Lens

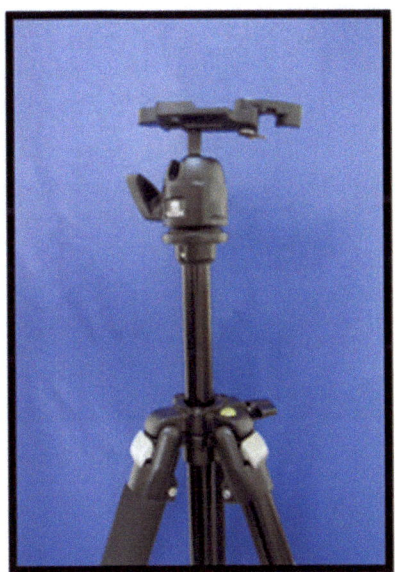

Figure 2.3: Height adjustable tripod.

CHAPTER TWO
Materials and Methods

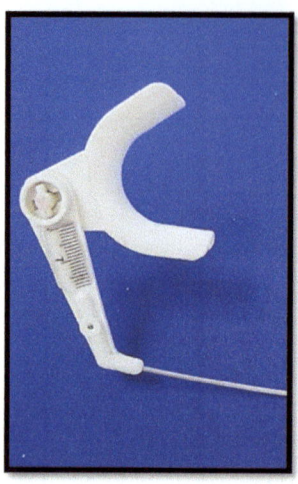 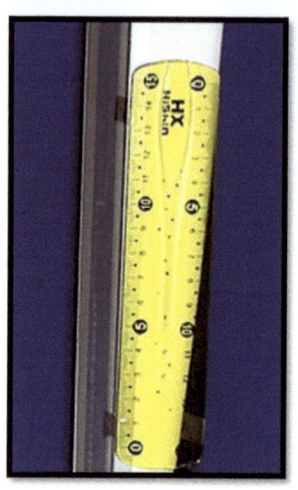

Figure 2.4: Ruler for intraoral photograph.   *Figure 2.5: Ruler for extraoral photograph.*

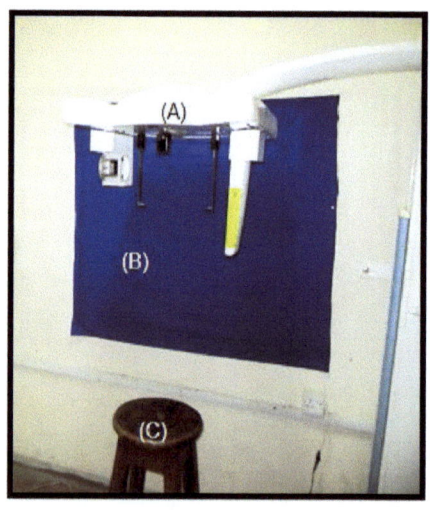

Figure 2.6: (A): Cephalostat, (B): Blue background, (C): Stool.

| CHAPTER TWO | Materials and Methods |

2.2. Methods
2.2.1. Ethical Consideration

Participants should be informed about the purpose of this study and that their photographs will be used for this research and may be used for future further investigations, any questions from the participants regarding the study were answered appropriately before enrolling in this study.

2.2.2. Clinical Examination
2.2.2.1. History

Each participant was seated on the dental chair and information about his/her name, age, medical and dental history was obtained from him/her, then each participant was examined clinically (extraoral and intraoral) to ensure his/her inclusion in the study according to criteria of sample selection. After that, a written consent form was obtained from the participants to assure their voluntary participation in the study. The case sheet for the clinical examination and the consent form were used in this study as shown in the appendix I, II.

2.2.2.2. Skeletal Examination

a. Anteroposterior Relation: each participant was postured in an upright position in dental chair with Frankfort plane parallel to the floor, and asked him/her to occlude gently on posterior teeth and gaze at a distant point **(Roberts-Harry and Sandy, 2003).**

As shown in **(Fig 2.7)**, by using the index finger of the right hand to palpate the soft tissue point A (deepest point in the upper lip at midline) and the middle finger to palpate the soft tissue point B (deepest point in the lower lip at midline), the skeletal pattern was assessed **(Foster, 1985).**

| CHAPTER TWO | Materials and Methods |

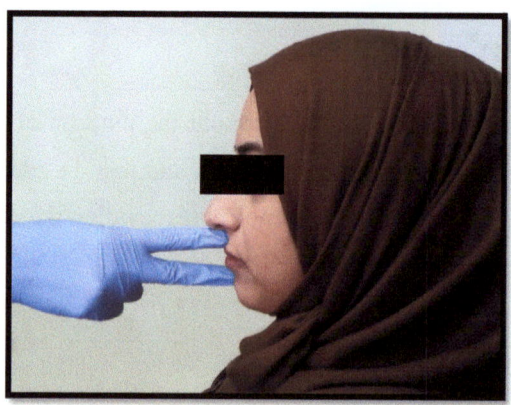

Figure 2.7: Assessment of anteroposterior relation by using Foster method.

b. Vertical Relation: The vertical relation was measured in terms of facial height, the upper anterior facial height was represented by the distance from the point between the eyebrows "glabella" to the base of the nose "subnasale", the lower anterior facial height was the distance from the soft tissue menton (base of the chin) to the base of the nose, after marking the points of glabella (Gl), subnasale (Sn), menton (Me) with a marker, the facial heights were measured with a vernier **(Roberts-Harry and Sandy, 2003)**, as shown in **(Fig 2.8).**

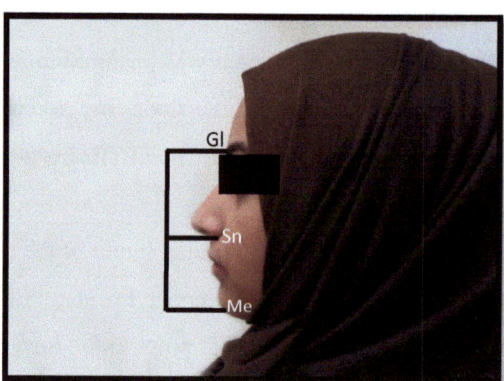

Figure 2.8: Measurement of upper and lower anterior facial heights, Gl: Glabella, Sn: Subnasale, Me: Menton.

c. Horizontal Relation: This dimension was assessed by looking at the participant head-on and assess whether there was asymmetry in the facial midline **(Roberts-Harry and Sandy, 2003).**

2.2.2.3. Dental Examination

Each participant was examined intraorally to ensure that all permanent teeth were present according to the previously mentioned criteria. Then the relation between the maxillary and mandibular teeth were examined:

a. Classification of Occlusion

-Molar Classification: In Class I normal occlusion, the tip of the mesio-buccal cusp of the maxillary first permanent molar should occlude with the mesio-buccal groove of the mandibular first permanent molar **(Angle, 1899, Foster, 1985; Sandeep and Sonia, 2012).**

-Canine Classification: The tip of maxillary permanent canine in Class I relation should occlude into the embrasure between the mandibular canine and mandibular first premolar **(Angle, 1899; Jones and Oliver, 2000).**

-Incisor classification: According to **British Standard Institution (BS4492, 1983)**, in Class I relation, the incisal edges of mandibular permanent incisors should occlude on or directly beneath the cingulum plateau of the maxillary permanent incisors.

b. Measurement of the Overjet and the Overbite

While the participant was in centric occlusion with his/ her occlusal plane horizontal, the overjet was measured with the use of dental vernier by placing the tip of vernier on the labial aspect of the mandibular central incisor, holding it against the incisal edge of the maxillary central incisor horizontally. The overjet was measured to the nearest millimeters **(Draker, 1960).**

Measurement of the overbite was made with the aid of a dental vernier, the amount of overlap of the maxillary incisors on the mandibular incisors was marked with the pencil on the labial aspect of the mandibular incisors, using the incisal edge of the maxillary incisor to guide the pencil, the upper conical plane of the sharpened part of the pencil and not the shaft of the pencil itself was placed parallel to the participant's occlusal plane, the measurement from the incisal edge of the mandibular central incisor to the pencil mark was made to the nearest millimeter **(Draker, 1960; Baume *et al.*, 1973).**

c. In addition to the classification of occlusion and measurements of the overjet and overbite, the presence of spacing or crowding, posterior crossbite, signs of gingival or periodontal diseases were assessed clinically according to the criteria of sample selection.

2.2.3. Standardization of the Photographs

The camera fixed in position and adjusted in height to be at the level of the participant's eyes with a height adjustable tripod that controls the stability and the correct height of the camera according to the participant's body height. The distance from the camera to the participant was fixed at a distance of about 101 cm measured from the camera lens to the ear rods (**Meneghini, 2005**), the ear rods were fit in the external auditory meatus in order to avoid the forward, backward, and tilting of the subject head (Cephalostat based head position), **(Al-Ramahi, 2009)**, and 56 cm from the camera lens to the ear rods for frontal intraoral photographs **(Farias *et al.*, 2010)**. The EF-S 18-200mm f/3.5-5.6 IS lens was used, participants were seated on a constant chair in front of a blue background which was made from a piece of cloth, as shown in **(Fig 2.9, 2.10, 2.11)**

CHAPTER TWO

Materials and Methods

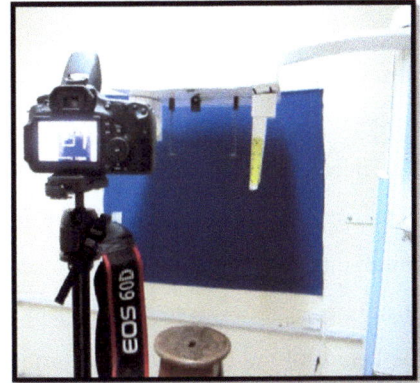 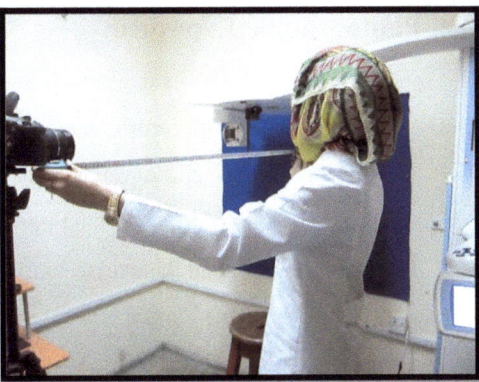

Figure 2.9: The camera fixed in position with a height adjustable tripod.

Figure 2.10: The distance between the subjects and the camera lens measured with measuring tap.

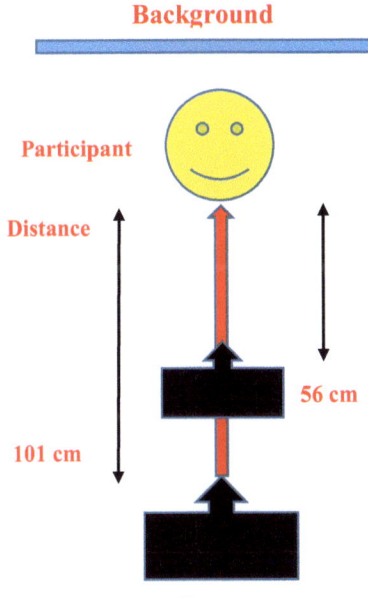

Figure 2.11: The distance between the subjects and the camera lens was 56 cm for intraoral photograph and 101cm for extraoral photograph.

2.2.4. Photographic Exposure

Two photographs (Frontal facial and intraoral photographs) were taken with the participant closed in centric occlusion.

For the facial photographs, each participant was positioned in the cephalostat with the interpupillary plane parallel to the floor **(Aksakalli and Demir, 2013)**, and instructed to keep their teeth in maximum intercuspation and gently closed lips **(Asghari *et al.*, 2014)**. The camera lens positioned parallel to the participant's face and the participant was asked to look at the center of the camera's lens during taking the photograph with the participant's hair did not cover any part of the face **(Wolfart *et al.*, 2004; Varjão *et al.*, 2006)** as shown in **(Fig 2.12)**, a ruler was placed on the plastic side of cephalostat near the participant's head to correct the magnification.

For intraoral photograph, the cheek retractor was used to clearly display maxillary anterior teeth, with the camera lens parallel to the labial surface of the teeth **(Koralakunte and Budihal, 2012)**. A piece of a ruler was attached to the retractor to correct the magnification.

2.2.5. The Digital Camera Set-Up

The digital camera was set on the manual exposure shooting chosen from the model dial that determined the desired function. From the wheel dial the camera was set on the following setting *(depending on the lighting level of the photographing room and with aid of specialist):*

- ✓ ISO (International Standardization Organization) which refers to the level of sensitivity of the digital camera to the available light, set on value of **2000**.
- ✓ Shutter speed which refers to the length of time that the camera shutter was opened to expose light into the camera sensor, set on **80** (which means 1/80 of a second).

| CHAPTER TWO | Materials and Methods |

- ✓ Aperture value which refers to the diameter of the lens hole through which the light travels to the camera body, set on **f/5.6**.
- ✓ Flash **on**.

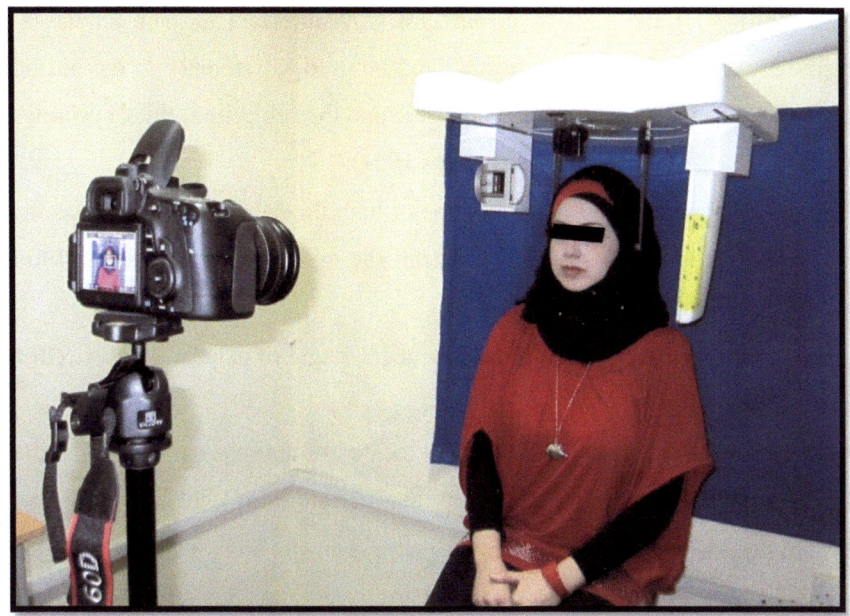

Figure 2.12: Participant was positioned in the cephalostat and instructed to look at the center of the camera's lens during taking the photograph.

2.2.6. Photographic Analysis

Each frontal facial and intraoral photographs was analyzed by AutoCAD 2014 program. Once the picture was imported to the AutoCAD program, it appeared in the master sheet on which the points were located then the measurements (extraoral and intraoral) were determined. The measurements were divided by scale for each picture to overcome the magnification.

2.2.6.1. The Macro-aesthetic Appearance

a. Facial Landmarks: Fig (2.13)

- **Glabella (Gl):** It is the most prominent point on the midline of the face, between the eyebrows, if the glabella is not clearly visible and the subject has a thin eyebrows, the top border of eyebrows can be used as reference to the position of the glabella and if the glabella is not visible and the subject has thick eyebrows, the middle of eyebrows can be used **(Farkas 1994).**
- **Nasion (n):** It is the point in the midline of both the nasal root and the nasofrontal suture, always above the line that connects the two inner canthi, identical to bone nasion **(Farkas et al., 1994).**
- **Inner canthus of the eye (Ic):** It is the medial angle of palpebral fissure **(Bishara et al., 1995).**
- **Pupil's of the eye (p):** It is the hole that located in the center of the iris of the eye that allows light to enter the retina **(Cassin and Solomon, 1990).**
- **Zygoin (zy):** It is most lateral point on each zygomatic arch, widest part of the face below the level of the eyes **(Gosman, 1950).**
- **Alare of the nose (AL):** It is located at each lateral rim of the ala of the nose at its widest width **(Gosman, 1950).**
- **Subnasale (Sn):** It is the point at which the nasal columella merges with upper mucocutaneous lip in the mid sagittal plane **(Powell and Humphreys, 1984).**
- **Chilion (Ch):** It is a point located at each angle of the mouth and selected to be on the same level with stomion **(Ricketts, 1982).**
- **Stomion (Sto):** It is the midpoint of the intra-labial fissure **(Milutinovic et al., 2014).**
- **The Labrale Superius (LS):** The midpoint in the upper margin of the upper membranous lip **(Bishara, 2001).**
- **The Labrale Inferius (LI):** The midpoint in the lower margin of the lower membranous lip **(Bishara, 2001).**

CHAPTER TWO   Materials and Methods

- **Menton (Me):** It is a point located at the lower border of the soft tissue chin **(Bell et al., 1986)**.

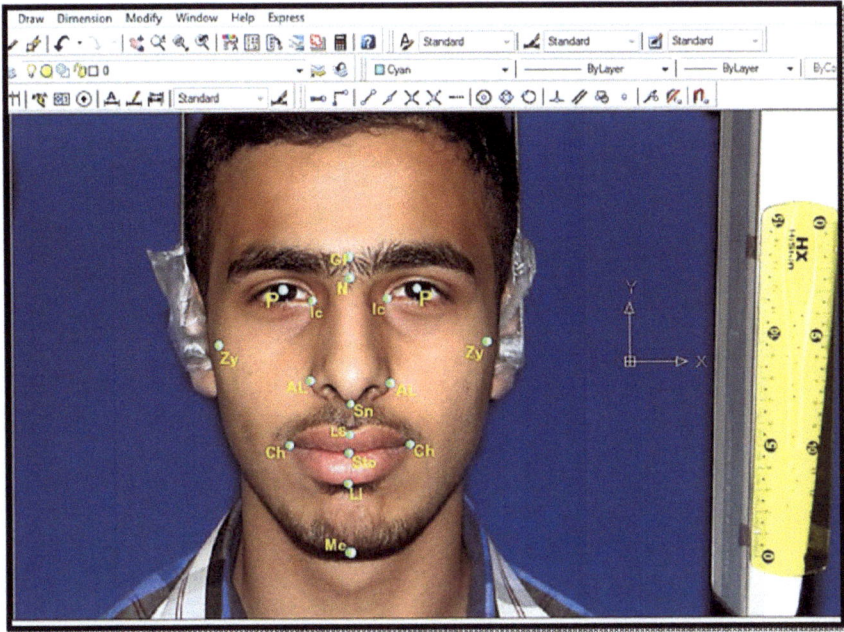

Figure 2.13: Facial Landmarks, Gl: Glabella, N: Nasion, Ic: Inner canthus of the eye, P: Pupil's of the eye, Zy: Zygoin, AL: Alare of the nose, Sn: Subnasale, Ch: Chilion, Sto: Stomion, LS: The Labrale Superius, LI: The Labrale Inferius, Me: Menton.

b. The Horizontal Facial Measurements: as shown in **(Fig 2.14)**

- **Zygomatic width (zy-zy):** The distance between the two zygion points **(Farkas, 1986)**.
- **Inter-canthal distance (ICD):** The distance between the median (inner) angles (canthi) of the palpebral fissure **(Al-Wazzan, 2001)**.
- **Interpupillary width (IPW):** It is a horizontal line that connects between the center of right and left pupils **(Haraguchia et al., 2008)**.
- **Interalar width (IAW):** The distance between the outer points of the ala of the nose **(Gomes et al., 2009)**.

- **Mouth width (MW):** The distance between the two angles of the mouth, from chilion to chilion **(Ricketts, 1982)**.

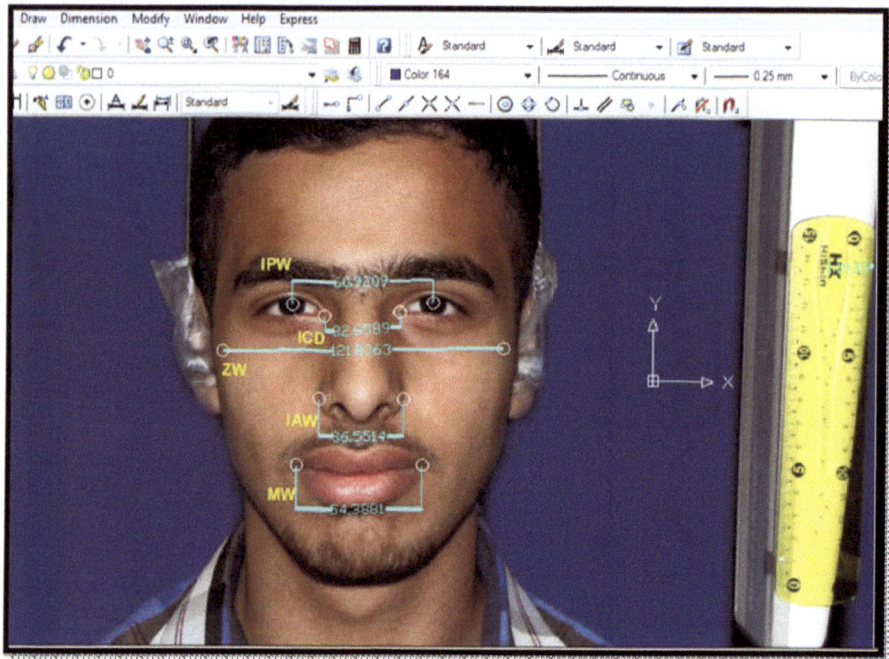

Figure 2.14: The Linear Facial Measurements, IPW: Interpupillary width, ICD: Inter-canthal distance, ZW: Zygomatic width, IAW: Interalar width, MW: Mouth width.

c. **The Vertical Facial Measurements:** as shown in **(Fig 2.15)**

- **Facial height (FH):** The distance between the soft tissue nasion and menton **(Ramadan, 2000)**.
- **Lower face height (LFH):** The distance between the subnasale and menton.
- **Upper lip vermilion (ULV):** The distance between labrale superius and stomion **(Bishara et al., 1995)**.
- **Lower lip vermilion (LLV):** The. distance between labrale inferius and stomion **(Bishara et al., 1995)**.

| CHAPTER TWO | Materials and Methods |

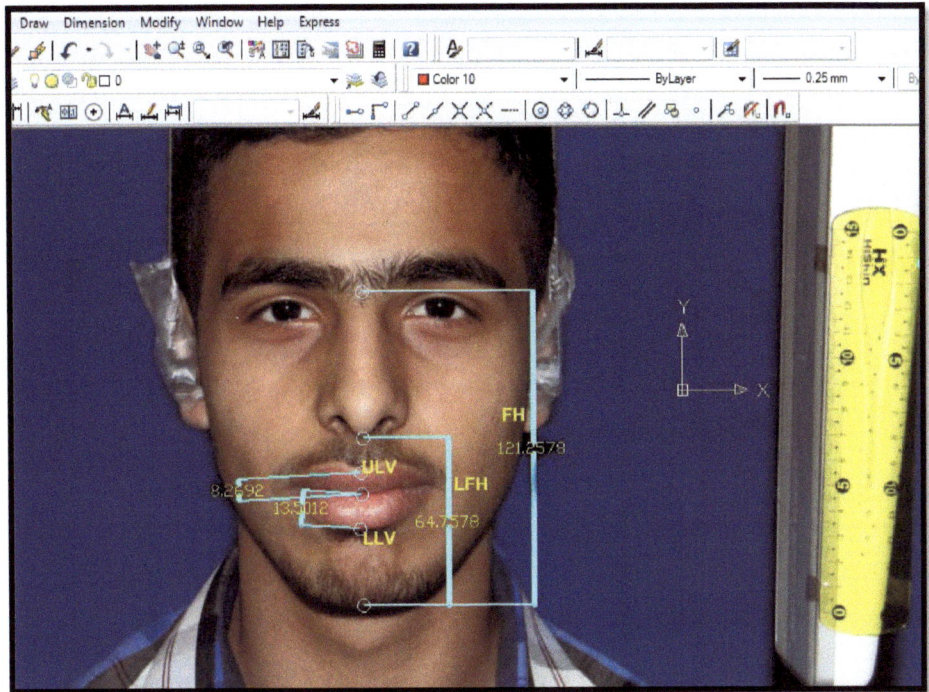

Figure 2.15: Vertical Facial Measurements, N-Me: Facial height, ULV: Upper lip vermilion, LLV: Lower lip vermilion, Gl-Sn: Middle third, Sn-Me: Lower third, Sn-Sto: subnasale-stomion, Sto-Me: stomion-menton.

2.2.6.2. The Micro-aesthetic Appearance

a. The Golden Proportion

The ratio of the recurring 62% proportions, for each participant was measured so that, the width of the maxillary lateral incisor was 62% of the maxillary central incisor width and the width of the maxillary canine was 62% of the maxillary lateral incisor width **(Proffit *et al.*, 2013).** *The proportion of successive width of the teeth should remain constant when progressing distally from the midline* and it was calculated as follow:

CHAPTER TWO — Materials and Methods

- *The mesiodistal dimension* was measured parallel to the incisal edge, and at the widest mesio-distal portion of the tooth. **(Snow, 1999)**, as shown in **(Fig 2.16)**.

> *For the lateral incisor, the golden proportion* = MDW of lateral incisor * 100
>   MDW of central incisor

> *For the canine, the golden proportion* = MDW of canine * 100
>   MDW of lateral incisor

b. The Golden Percentage

The proportional width of each maxillary anterior tooth (for the right and left side) should be: **10%** for the canine, **15%** for the lateral incisor, **25%** for the central incisor of the total distance across the maxillary anterior segment, it was calculated as follow:

-*The mesiodistal dimension* measured at the widest mesio-distal portion of the tooth and parallel to the incisal edge of each central incisor, lateral incisor and parallel to the occlusal line for the canine **(Snow, 1999)**, as shown in **(Fig 2.16)**.

> *The golden percentage* = MDW of central, lateral, canine * 100
>   CMDW of all maxillary anterior teeth

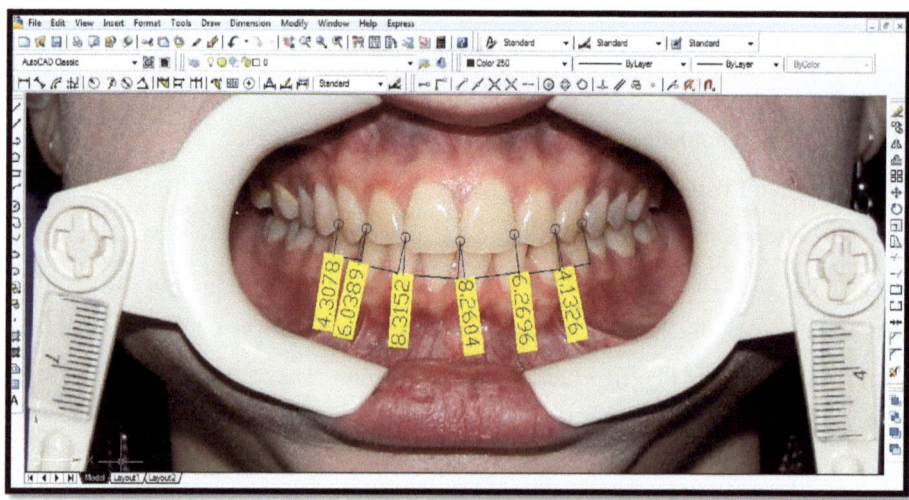

Figure 2.16: Measurement of mesiodistal width of maxillary anterior teeth.

c. Tooth Proportionality-Width and Height

The ideal maxillary central incisor should be approximately **80%** width compared to its height, but this ratio has been reported to vary between **66% and 80% (Gillen et al., 1994)**. It was calculated as follow:

-The incisogingival and mesiodistal dimensions of the maxillary central incisor were measured at the longest apico-coronal portion of the tooth and widest mesio-distal portion **(Zlataric et al., 2007)**, as shown in **(Fig 2.17)**.

> *Width/height ratio* = $\dfrac{\textit{Width of the tooth}}{\textit{Height of the tooth}} * 100$

d. Height of Contact Points

Contacts between the maxillary anterior teeth were where the teeth actually touch **(Sarver, 2004)**. The golden ratio was applied to the height of contact points of the anterior teeth. The contact points between the maxillary central incisors should correspond to **50%** of the height of the crown of these teeth, and should gradually distally reduce, turning into **40%** of this height at the contact point between the maxillary central and lateral incisors, and **30%** of this height at the contact point between the maxillary lateral incisor and the canine, this ratio was calculated as follow:

-The height of contact point was measured from the incisal convergence of the gingival embrasure to the gingival convergence of the incisal embrasure **(Morley and Eubank, 2001)**, as shown in **(Fig 2.17)**.

> *For central incisor* = $\dfrac{\textit{Height of contact point between centrals}}{\textit{Height of central incisor}} * 100$

> *For lateral incisor* = $\dfrac{\textit{Height of contact point between central and lateral}}{\textit{Height of central incisor}} * 100$

> *For canine* = $\dfrac{\textit{Height of contact point between lateral and canine}}{\textit{Height of central incisor}} * 100$

- Total Maxillary Anterior Teeth Width

The distance between the tips of the maxillary canines in a horizontal straight line was measured **(Gomes *et al.*, 2009)**, as shown in **(Fig 2.17)**.

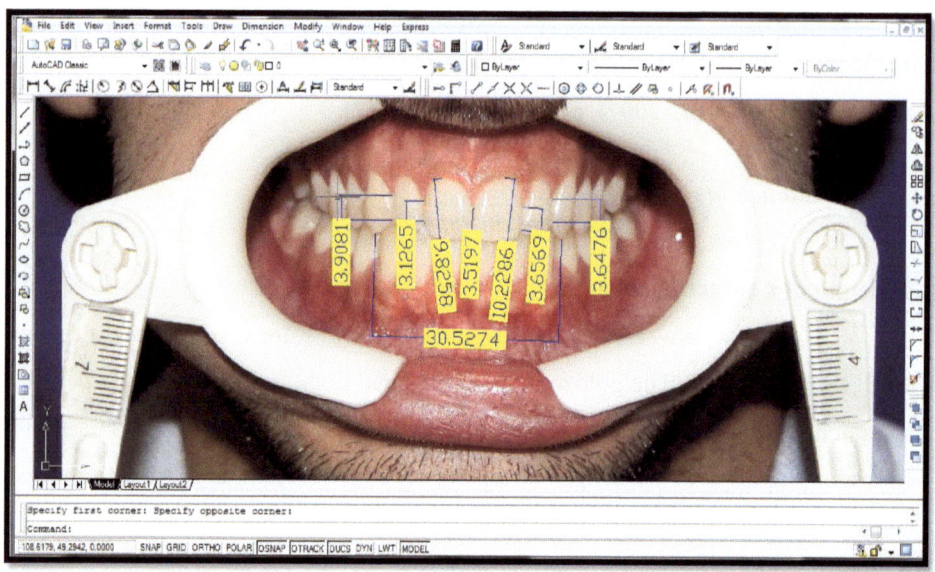

Figure 2.17: Measurement of the height of maxillary central incisors, height of contact points and total maxillary anterior teeth width.

2.3. Pilot Study

According to *van Teijlingen and Hundley (2002)*, the term 'pilot study' refers to the mini versions of a full-scale study and the specific pre-testing of a particular research instruments, it does not guarantee the success in the main research but it does increase the liklihood of success. So before starting the required measurements, the pilot study was conducted on a randomly selected 10 photographs (extraoral and intraoral) used in this research work to assess the reliability and accuracy of the measurements, the following tests were taken:

CHAPTER TWO — Materials and Methods

a. Inter-examiner calibration, where importing photographs to the Autocad software, correction of the magnification, landmarks identification and measurements were carried out by professional examiner (orthodontist) for the selected records. Table (2.1, 2.2)

Table 2.1: Inter-examiner calibration of the facial measurements.

Variables	Descriptive statistics				Readings difference			
	Professional reading		Researcher reading		Mean difference	t-test	p-value	Sig
	Mean	S.D.	Mean	S.D.				
ICD	34.39	3.01	34.19	3.14	0.20	2.112	0.088	
IPD	64.67	3.07	64.42	2.98	0.25	1.847	0.124	
zy-zy	131.31	8.48	131.32	8.24	-0.01	-0.103	0.922	
IAW	39.80	3.76	39.85	3.65	-0.05	-0.395	0.709	
MW	53.32	3.19	53.40	3.12	-0.08	-1.021	0.354	NS
FH	128.08	12.19	128.03	12.23	0.05	0.903	0.408	
LFH	66.72	10.98	66.41	10.95	0.31	2.114	0.088	
ULV	5.49	0.67	5.37	0.59	0.12	1.157	0.300	
LLV	10.22	2.00	10.25	2.17	-0.03	-0.266	0.801	

*N=10, d.f = 9, all measurements were in mm. NS: Non-Significant difference (P > 0.05)

Table 2.2: Inter-examiner calibration of intraoral measurements.

Variables	Descriptive statistics				Readings difference			
	Professional reading		Researcher reading		Mean Difference	t-test	p-value	Sig
	Mean	S.D.	Mean	S.D.				
MDW CI (Left)	8.43	0.53	8.52	0.46	-0.09	-2.566	0.051	
Height of CI (Left)	10.08	1.00	10.00	1.00	0.08	1.526	0.188	
MDW CI (Right)	8.30	0.62	8.38	0.58	-0.08	-1.407	0.218	
Height of CI (Right)	10.01	0.99	10.02	0.87	-0.01	-0.121	0.908	
MDW LI (Left)	5.77	0.76	5.79	0.70	-0.02	-0.277	0.793	
MDW LI (Right)	5.66	0.69	5.65	0.79	0.01	0.148	0.888	
MDW Ca (Left)	4.92	0.32	4.89	0.45	0.03	0.357	0.736	NS
MDW Ca (Right)	4.65	0.38	4.64	0.40	0.01	0.223	0.832	
ICaD	33.42	1.52	33.06	1.73	0.36	2.178	0.081	
Height of contact point CI-CI	3.65	0.51	3.68	0.50	-0.03	-0.561	0.599	
Height of contact point Left CI-LI	3.20	1.16	3.09	1.04	0.11	1.206	0.282	
Height of contact point Right CI-LI	3.53	0.46	3.42	0.61	0.11	0.763	0.480	
Height of contact point Left LI-Ca	2.60	0.58	2.50	0.75	0.10	1.258	0.264	
Height of contact point Right LI-Ca	2.83	0.49	2.78	0.52	0.05	0.847	0.436	

*N= 10, d.f = 9, all measurements were in mm. NS: Non-Significant difference (P > 0.05)

b. **Intra-examiner calibration**, where the landmarks identification and measurements carried out twice by the same researcher, with two weeks interval between the two measurements to avoid the memory bias. Table (2.3, 2.4)

Table 2.3: Intra-examiner calibration of the facial measurements.

Variables	Descriptive statistics				Readings difference			
	1st reading		2nd reading		Mean Difference	t-test	p-value	Sig
	Mean	S.D.	Mean	S.D.				
ICD	34.19	3.14	34.22	3.28	-0.03	-0.240	0.820	
IPD	64.42	2.98	64.13	2.72	0.29	1.885	0.118	
zy-zy	131.32	8.24	131.26	8.35	0.06	0.472	0.657	
IAW	39.85	3.65	40.06	3.84	-0.21	-1.640	0.162	
MW	53.40	3.12	53.45	3.02	-0.05	-0.731	0.497	NS
FH	128.03	12.23	128.01	12.16	0.02	0.329	0.755	
LFH	66.41	10.95	66.42	11.03	-0.01	-0.084	0.937	
ULV	5.37	0.59	5.40	0.64	-0.03	-0.397	0.708	
LLV	10.25	2.17	10.36	1.89	-0.11	-0.704	0.513	

*N= 10, d.f= 9, all measurements were in mm. NS: Non-Significant difference (P > 0.05).

Table 2.4: Intra-examiner calibration of intraoral measurements.

Variables	Descriptive statistics				Readings difference			
	1st reading		2nd reading		Mean Difference	t-test	p-value	Sig
	Mean	S.D.	Mean	S.D.				
MDW CI (Left)	8.52	0.46	8.53	0.45	-0.01	-0.331	0.754	
Height of CI (Left)	10.00	1.00	9.94	1.01	0.06	2.040	0.097	
MDW CI (Right)	8.38	0.58	8.39	0.54	-0.01	-0.500	0.639	
Height of CI (Right)	10.02	0.87	10.03	0.87	-0.01	-0.233	0.825	
MDW LI (Left)	5.79	0.70	5.84	0.75	-0.05	-0.966	0.379	
MDW LI (Right)	5.65	0.79	5.65	0.75	0.00	-0.134	0.899	
MDW Ca (Left)	4.89	0.45	4.93	0.45	-0.04	-0.862	0.428	
MDW Ca (Right)	4.64	0.40	4.65	0.41	-0.01	-0.264	0.803	NS
ICaD	33.06	1.73	33.13	1.60	-0.07	-0.791	0.465	
Height of contact point CI-CI	3.68	0.50	3.68	0.53	0.00	-0.026	0.981	
Height of contact point Left CI-LI	3.09	1.04	3.04	1.10	0.05	0.737	0.494	
Height of contact point Right CI-LI	3.42	0.61	3.37	0.73	0.05	0.887	0.416	
Height of contact point Left LI-Ca	2.50	0.75	2.44	0.75	0.06	0.907	0.406	
Height of contact point Right LI-Ca	2.78	0.52	2.74	0.46	0.04	1.057	0.339	

*N= 10, d.f.= 9, all measurements were in mm. NS: Non-Significant difference (P > 0.05).

CHAPTER TWO Materials and Methods

2.4 Statistical Analysis

All the data of the sample were subjected to computerized statistical analysis using SPSS (statistical package of social science) software version 19. The statistical analysis included the followings:

1. Descriptive Statistics

a) Mean.

b) Standard deviation (SD).

c) Statistical tables and figures.

2. Inferential Statistics

a) Paired samples t-test: for intra- and inter-examiner calibrations and for side difference of the micro-aesthetic appearance.

b) Independent samples t-test: for the comparison between both genders.

c) Pearson's correlation coefficients (r): used to test the relationships between the measured variables in both genders.

In the statistical evaluation, the following levels of significance were used:

- $P > 0.05$ Non-significant.
- $0.05 \geq P > 0.01$ Significant.
- $P \leq 0.01$ Highly significant.

In the statistical evaluation, the following levels determine the strength of the relationship:

- $0.7 \leq |r| \leq 1.0$ the correlation is strong.
- $0.3 \leq |r| \leq 0.7$ the correlation is moderate.
- $|r| < 0.3$ the correlation is weak.

In the statistical evaluation, the following signs determine the type of the relationship:

- (+) r   the correlation is direct.
- (-) r   the correlation is indirect.

CHAPTER THREE — Results

Results

3.1. Sample

The sample of this study consisted of 120 participants (60 males and 60 females) from College of Dentistry-University of Baghdad, the age of the participants ranged between 18-23 years and the mean age of the participants was 21 years, as shown in table 3.1.

Table 3.1: The sample of this study and their mean age.

	The sample (120 individuals)	
Gender	Males	Females
	60 (50%)	60 (50%)
Mean age	21 years	

3.2. Descriptive Statistics and Gender Differences in Macro-aesthetic Appearance

Table 3.2 and Fig (3.1) indicated that the mean values of all measured variables were higher in males than females *except* in the upper (ULV) and lower lip vermilion (LLV) which were higher in females than males.

Independent sample t-test in table 3.2 indicated that there was a high significant difference regarding the Interpupillary width (IPW), Interalar width (IAW), Mouth width (MW), Facial height (FH), Lower face height (LFH) and non-significant gender difference in the Inter-canthal distance (ICD), Zygomatic width (zy-zy), Upper lip vermilion (ULV), and Lower lip vermilion (LLV).

CHAPTER THREE — Results

Table 3.2: Descriptive statistics and gender differences in macro-aesthetic appearance for male and female groups.

Variables	Descriptive statistics				Gender difference (d.f.= 118)		
	Males (N=60)		Females (N=60)		Mean Difference	t-test	p-value
	Mean	S.D.	Mean	S.D.			
ICD	31.62	3.17	30.89	3.37	0.73	1.230	0.221 (NS)
IPW	63.41	4.69	60.96	4.59	2.45	2.888	0.005 (HS)
zy-zy	127.77	7.68	125.73	9.05	2.04	1.334	0.185 (NS)
IAW	39.68	3.07	35.51	3.26	4.18	7.225	0.000 (HS)
MW	52.54	3.78	49.58	4.56	2.96	3.872	0.000 (HS)
FH	125.60	9.02	115.47	7.95	10.13	6.524	0.000 (HS)
LFH	69.92	5.23	60.63	5.43	9.29	9.537	0.000 (HS)
ULV	5.33	1.29	5.38	1.02	-0.05	-0.216	0.829 (NS)
LLV	10.11	1.76	10.29	1.48	-0.18	-0.617	0.538 (NS)

All measurements were in mm. NS: Non-Significant difference, S: Significant, HS: Highly Significant

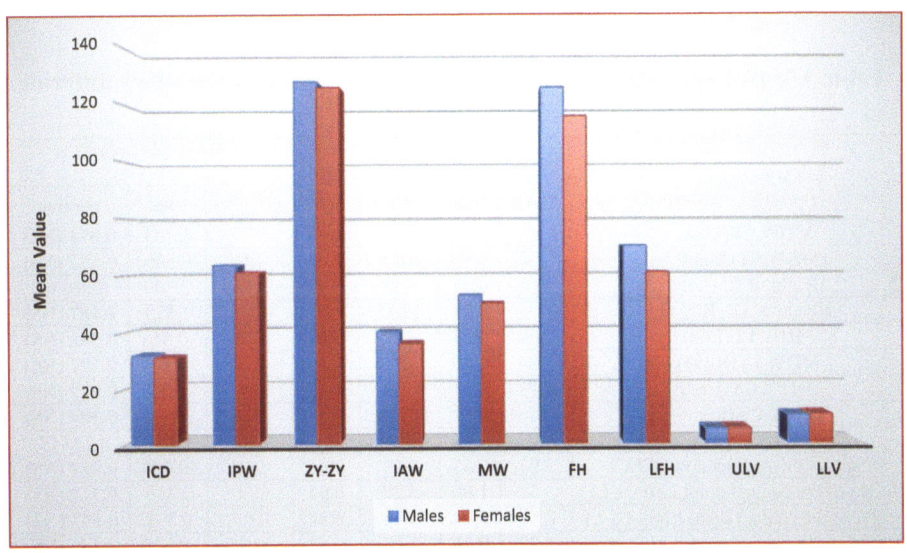

Figure 3.1: Descriptive statistics and gender differences in macro-aesthetic appearance for male and female groups.

CHAPTER THREE — Results

3.3. Descriptive Statistics and Gender Differences in Maxillary Anterior Teeth Variables

Table 3.3 and Fig (3.2) showed that the mean values of all measured variables were higher in males than females *except* in the mesiodistal width of the left and right lateral incisor (MDW LI), height of the contact point between "central incisors (CI-CI), lateral incisor and canine (left and right LI-Ca)", whereas the mean values of mesiodistal width of left canine (MDW Ca) were equal in both genders.

Additionally, the independent sample t-test in table 3.3 revealed a non-significant difference regarding the maxillary anterior teeth variables *except* in the inter-canine distance (ICaD) where there was a high significant difference *and* the height of left central incisor (CI) and mesiodistal width of both central incisors (MDW CIs) where there were a significant gender differences.

Table 3.3: Descriptive statistics and gender differences in Maxillary anterior teeth variables.

Variables	Descriptive statistics				Gender difference (d.f.=118)		
	Males (N=60)		Females (N=60)		Mean difference	t-test	p-value
	Mean	S.D.	Mean	S.D.			
MDW CI (Left)	8.80	0.60	8.63	0.49	0.17	1.703	0.091 (NS)
MDW CI (Right)	10.37	0.96	10.26	1.06	0.11	0.596	0.552 (NS)
Height of CI (Left)	8.79	0.51	8.58	0.54	0.21	2.200	0.030 (S)
Height of CI (Right)	10.39	0.94	10.15	1.05	0.24	1.328	0.187 (NS)
MDW LI (Left)	5.84	0.53	5.90	0.64	-0.06	-0.554	0.581 (NS)
MDW LI (Right)	5.84	0.59	5.93	0.50	-0.09	-0.860	0.392 (NS)
MDW Ca (Left)	4.79	0.61	4.79	0.57	0.00	-0.028	0.977 (NS)
MDW Ca (Right)	4.70	0.61	4.59	0.54	0.11	1.032	0.304 (NS)
MDW CIs	17.59	1.08	17.21	1	0.38	2.009	0.047 (S)
Height of the contact point CI-CI	3.97	0.83	3.98	0.83	-0.01	-0.060	0.952 (NS)
Height of the contact point Left CI-LI	3.34	1.00	3.28	0.94	0.06	0.363	0.717 (NS)
Height of the contact point Right CI-LI	3.54	0.94	3.48	0.84	0.06	0.391	0.697 (NS)
Height of the contact point Left LI-Ca	2.92	0.86	3.00	0.88	-0.08	-0.529	0.598 (NS)
Height of the contact point Right LI-Ca	3.15	0.89	3.17	0.84	-0.02	-0.141	0.888 (NS)
IID	29.27	1.55	29.04	1.57	0.24	0.826	0.410 (NS)
ICaD	34.51	1.88	33.60	1.84	0.90	2.660	0.009 (HS)

All measurements were in mm. NS: Non-Significant difference, S: Significant, HS: Highly Significant

CHAPTER THREE

Results

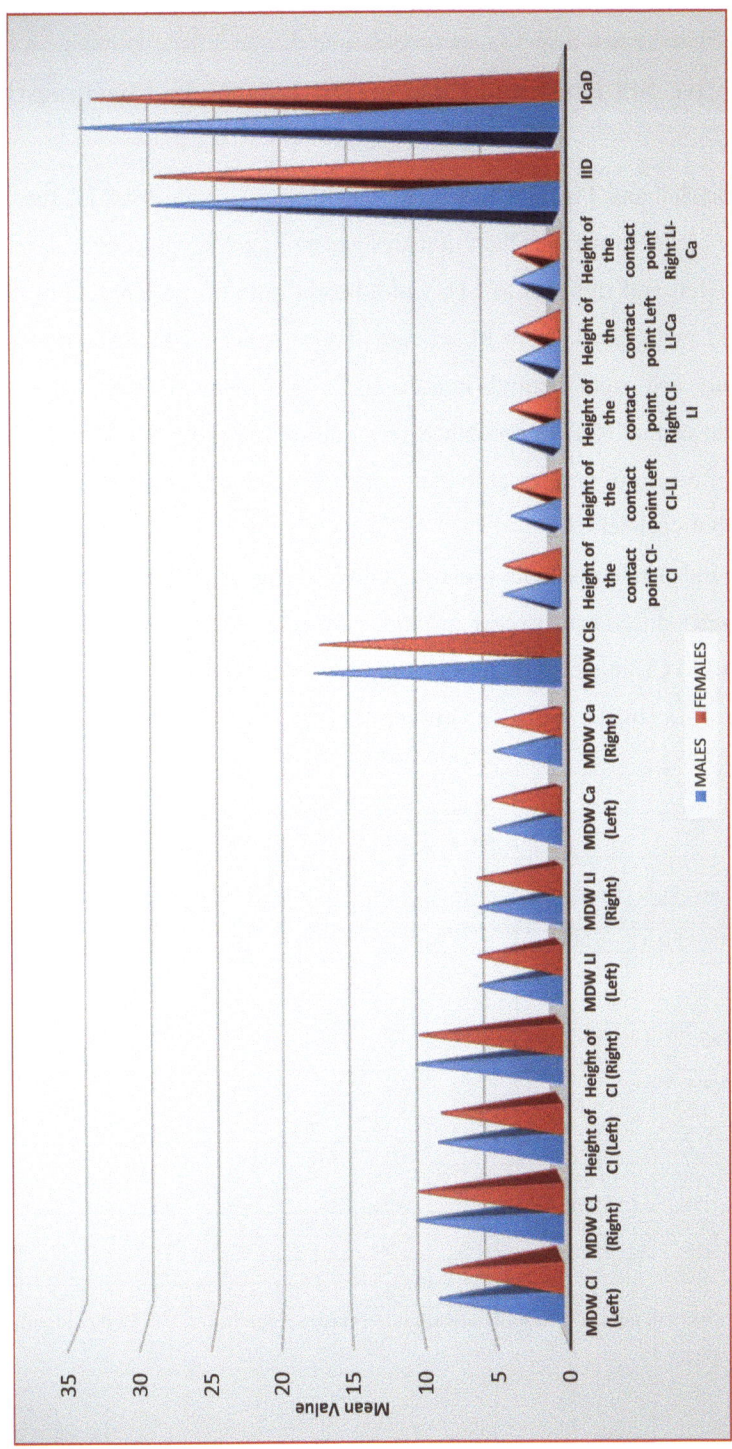

Figure 3.2: Descriptive statistics and gender differences in Maxillary anterior teeth variables.

CHAPTER THREE — Results

3.4. Descriptive Statistics and Gender Differences in Micro-aesthetic Appearance

Table 3.4 and Fig (3.3) revealed that the mean values of all measured variables were higher in females than in males *except* in golden proportion: canine to lateral incisor (left and right Ca to LI), width-height ratio of the left central incisor (CI), combined mesiodistal width of six maxillary anterior teeth (CMDW), golden percentage: left and right central incisors (CI) to combined mesiodistal width (CMDW), right canine (Ca) to combined mesiodistal width (CMDW), whereas the mean values of height of contact point % : central incisor-lateral incisor (left CI-LI) were equal in both genders.

The independent sample t-test in table 3.4 indicated the presence of a non-significant gender differences *except* in golden proportion: lateral incisor to central incisor (right LI to CI) in which there was a significant difference.

Table 3.4: Descriptive statistics and gender differences in micro-aesthetic appearance.

Variables	Descriptive statistics				Gender difference (d.f.=118)		
	Males (N=60)		Females (N=60)		Mean Difference	t-test	p-value
	Mean	S.D.	Mean	S.D.			
Golden proportion: Left LI to CI	66.71	7.68	68.53	7.83	-1.82	-1.287	0.201 (NS)
Golden proportion: Right LI to CI	66.55	6.68	69.29	6.46	-2.74	-2.284	0.024 (S)
Golden proportion: Left Ca to LI	82.55	12.25	81.91	11.42	0.64	0.297	0.767 (NS)
Golden proportion: Right Ca to LI	80.95	11.45	77.96	11.27	2.99	1.441	0.152 (NS)
Width-height ratio of left CI	85.41	7.72	84.91	8.90	0.50	0.328	0.743 (NS)
Width-height ratio of right CI	85.07	7.16	85.21	8.70	-0.14	-0.099	0.921 (NS)
CMDW	38.76	2.07	38.42	1.97	0.34	0.926	0.356 (NS)
Golden percentage: left CI to CMDW	22.72	1.23	22.48	1.02	0.24	1.150	0.252 (NS)
Golden percentage: right CI to CMDW	22.69	1.02	22.33	1.02	0.36	1.927	0.056 (NS)
Golden percentage: left LI to CMDW	15.09	1.23	15.35	1.30	-0.26	-1.141	0.256 (NS)
Golden percentage: right LI to CMDW	15.05	1.18	15.43	1.10	-0.37	-1.794	0.075 (NS)
Golden percentage: left Ca to CMDW	12.35	1.33	12.47	1.24	-0.12	-0.521	0.603 (NS)
Golden percentage: right Ca to CMDW	12.10	1.34	11.94	1.24	0.17	0.707	0.481 (NS)
Height of contact point %: CI-CI (left)	38.27	6.95	38.80	6.95	-0.52	-0.412	0.681 (NS)
Height of contact point %: CI-CI (right)	38.18	6.90	39.19	6.95	-1.01	-0.800	0.425 (NS)
Height of contact point % : CI-LI (left)	32.03	8.54	32.03	8.73	0	0	1 (NS)
Height of contact point % : CI-LI (right)	33.93	7.80	34.38	7.85	-0.45	-0.315	0.754 (NS)
Height of contact point % : LI-Ca (left)	27.96	7.41	29.26	8.20	-1.30	-0.912	0.364 (NS)
Height of contact point % : LI-Ca (right)	30.13	7.49	31.19	7.19	-1.05	-0.785	0.434 (NS)

All measurements were in mm. NS: Non-Significant difference, S: Significant, HS: Highly Significant

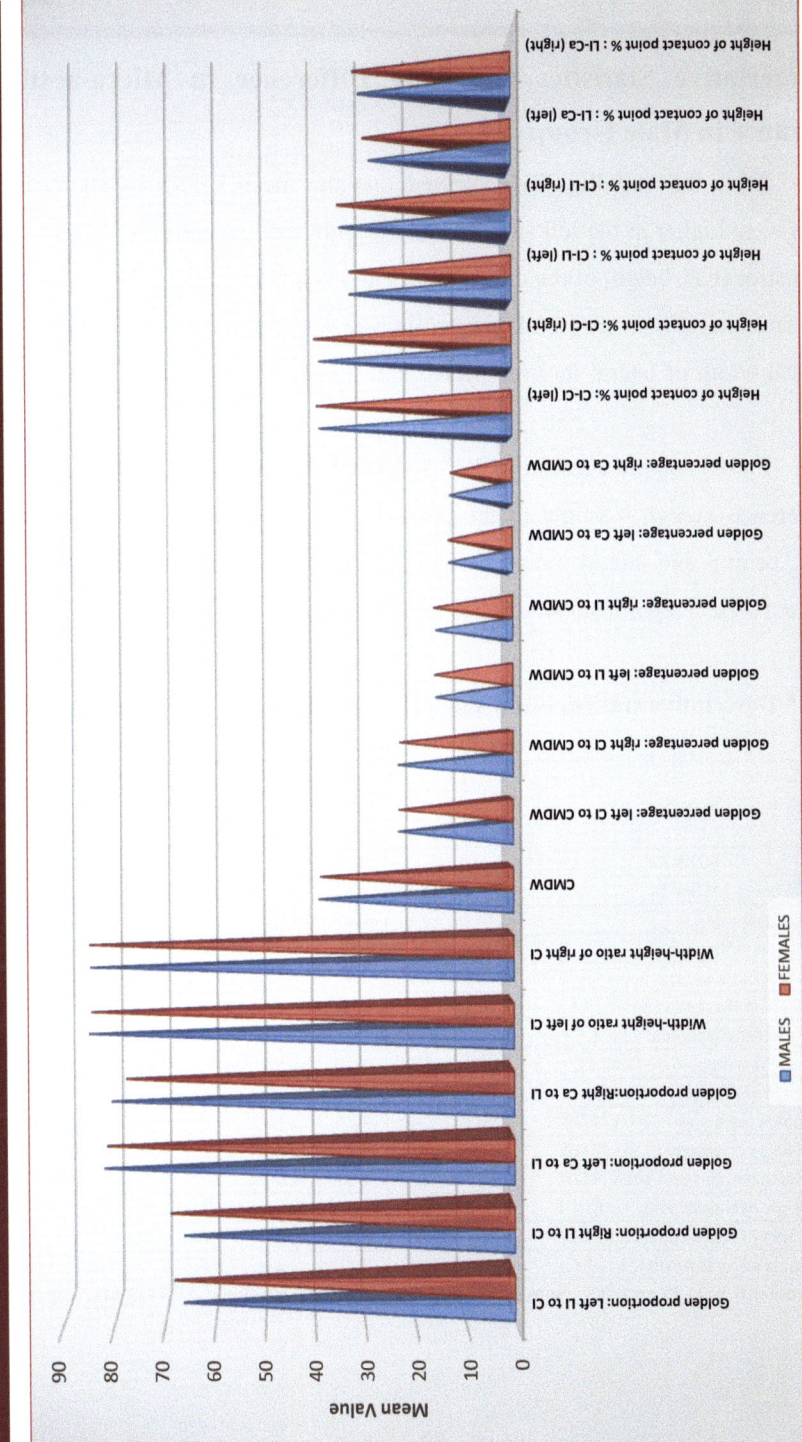

Figure 3.3: Descriptive statistics and gender differences in micro-aesthetic appearance.

CHAPTER THREE — Results

3.5. Descriptive Statistics and Side Difference in Micro-aesthetic Appearance in Male Group

Table 3.5 and Fig (3.4) showed that the mean values of all measured variables were higher in the left side than in the right side *except* in the height of the central incisor (CI), height of the contact point and height of contact point % between "central and lateral incisor (CI-LI), lateral incisor and canine (LI-Ca)", and only in mesiodistal width of lateral incisor (MDW LI), the mean values were equal in both sides.

Paired sample t-test in table 3.5 showed that there was a non-significant side difference *except* in height of the contact point and height of the contact point % between "central and lateral incisor (CI-LI), lateral incisor and canine (LI-Ca)", in which there were a significant side differences.

Table 3.5 Descriptive statistics and side difference in micro-aesthetic appearance in male group.

Variables	Descriptive statistics				Side difference (d.f.= 59)		
	Left side		Right side				
	Mean	S.D.	Mean	S.D.	MD	t-test	p-value
MDW CI	8.80	0.60	8.79	0.51	0.01	0.399	**0.691 (NS)**
MDW LI	**5.84**	0.53	**5.84**	0.59	0.00	0.053	**0.958 (NS)**
MDW Ca	4.79	0.61	4.70	0.61	0.10	1.039	**0.303 (NS)**
Height of CI	10.37	0.96	10.39	0.94	-0.02	-0.527	**0.600 (NS)**
Height of the contact point: CI-LI	3.34	1.00	3.54	0.94	-0.20	-2.359	**0.022 (S)**
Height of the contact point: LI-Ca	2.92	0.86	3.15	0.89	-0.23	-2.583	**0.012 (S)**
Golden proportion: LI to CI	66.71	7.68	66.55	6.68	0.16	0.193	**0.847 (NS)**
Golden proportion: Ca to LI	82.55	12.25	80.95	11.45	1.60	0.911	**0.366 (NS)**
Width-height ratio of CI	85.41	7.72	85.07	7.16	0.34	0.802	**0.426 (NS)**
Golden percentage: CI to CMDW	22.72	1.23	22.69	1.02	0.03	0.336	**0.738 (NS)**
Golden percentage: LI to CMDW	15.09	1.23	15.05	1.18	0.03	0.166	**0.869 (NS)**
Golden percentage: Ca to CMDW	12.35	1.33	12.10	1.34	0.24	1.019	**0.312 (NS)**
Height of contact point % : CI-CI	38.27	6.95	38.18	6.90	0.09	0.587	**0.560 (NS)**
Height of contact point % : CI-LI	32.03	8.54	33.93	7.80	-1.90	-2.268	**0.027 (S)**
Height of contact point % : LI-Ca	27.96	7.41	30.13	7.49	-2.18	-2.551	**0.013 (S)**

All measurements were in mm. NS: Non-Significant difference, S: Significant, HS: Highly Significant

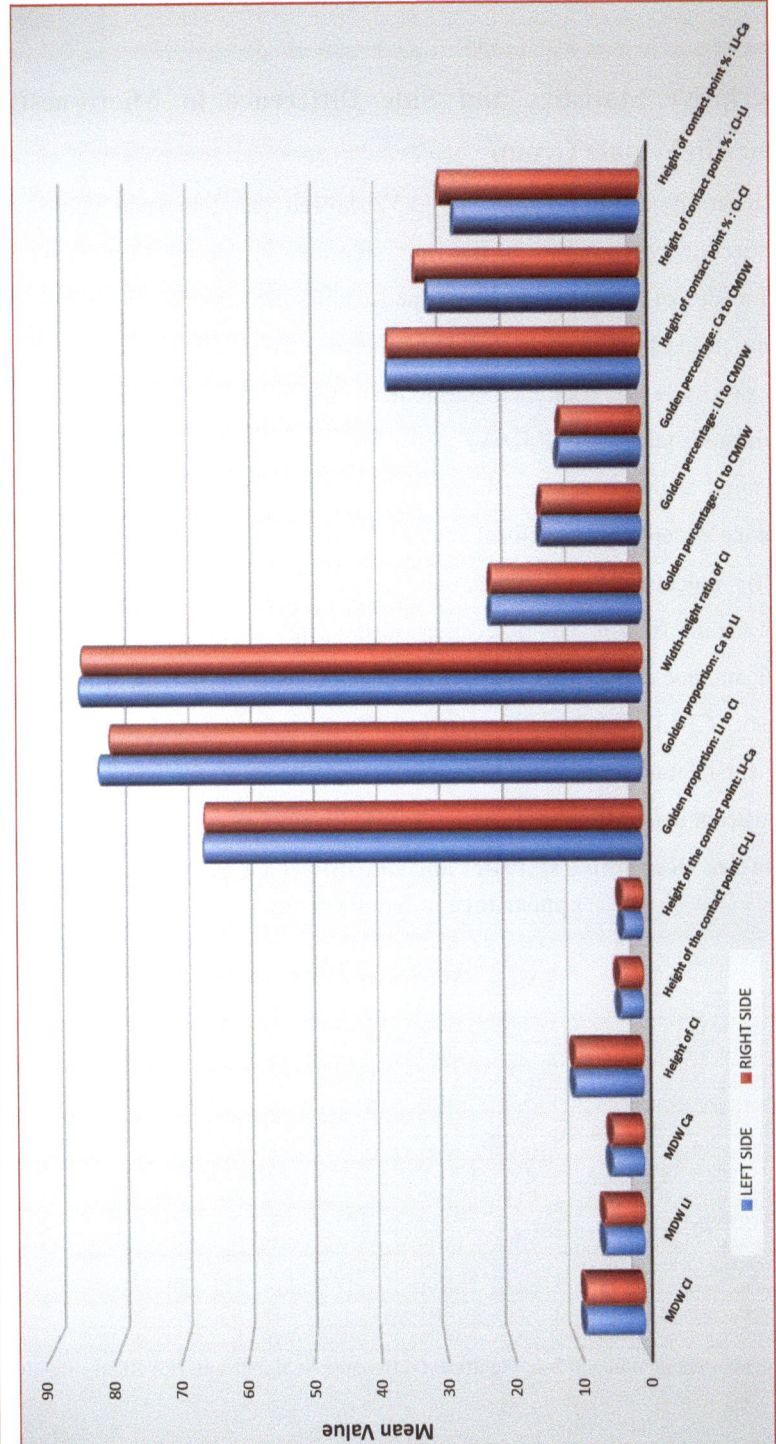

Figure 3.4: Descriptive statistics and side difference in micro-aesthetic appearance in male group.

3.6. Descriptive Statistics and Side Difference in Micro-aesthetic Appearance in Female Group

Generally, table 3.6 and Fig (3.5) showed that the mean values of all measured variables were higher in the right side than in the left side *except* in the mesiodistal width of central incisor (CI) and canine (Ca), height of central incisor (CI), golden proportion: canine to lateral incisor (CI to LI), golden percentage: central incisor (CI) to combined mesiodistal width (CMDW), canine (Ca) to combined mesiodistal width (CMDW).

Paired sample t-test in table 3.6 showed that there was a non-significant side difference except in mesiodistal width of canine (MDW Ca), height of central incisor (CI), golden proportion: canine to lateral incisor (Ca to LI), golden percentage: canine (Ca) to combined mesiodistal width (CMDW) which showed a high significant side differences, and height of the contact point between central and lateral incisor (CI-LI), height of contact point % between "central incisors (CI-CI), central incisor-lateral incisor (CI-LI), lateral incisor-canine (LI-Ca)", where there were a significant side differences.

Table 3.6: Descriptive statistics and side difference in micro-aesthetic appearance in female group.

Variables	Descriptive statistics				Side difference (d.f.= 59)		
	Left side		Right side		MD	t-test	p-value
	Mean	S.D.	Mean	S.D.			
MDW CI	8.63	0.49	8.58	0.54	0.06	1.674	0.099 (NS)
MDW LI	5.90	0.64	5.93	0.50	-0.02	-0.350	0.728 (NS)
MDW Ca	4.79	0.57	4.59	0.54	0.21	2.766	0.008 (HS)
Height of CI	10.26	1.06	10.15	1.05	0.11	2.684	0.009 (HS)
Height of the contact point: CI-LI	3.28	0.94	3.48	0.84	-0.20	-2.109	0.039 (S)
Height of the contact point: LI-Ca	3.00	0.88	3.17	0.84	-0.17	-1.778	0.080 (NS)
Golden proportion: LI to CI	68.53	7.83	69.29	6.46	-0.76	-0.957	0.343 (NS)
Golden proportion: Ca to LI	81.91	11.42	77.96	11.27	3.95	3.375	0.001 (HS)
Width-height ratio of CI	84.91	8.90	85.21	8.70	-0.30	-0.683	0.498 (NS)
Golden percentage: CI to CMDW	22.48	1.02	22.33	1.02	0.15	1.765	0.083 (NS)
Golden percentage: LI to CMDW	15.35	1.30	15.43	1.10	-0.08	-0.467	0.642 (NS)
Golden percentage: Ca to CMDW	12.47	1.24	11.94	1.24	0.53	2.776	0.007 (HS)
Height of contact point % : CI-CI	38.80	6.95	39.19	6.95	-0.40	-2.556	0.013 (S)
Height of contact point % : CI-LI	32.03	8.73	34.38	7.85	-2.34	-2.420	0.019 (S)
Height of contact point % : LI-Ca	29.26	8.20	31.19	7.19	-1.93	-2.155	0.035 (S)

All measurements were in mm. NS: Non-Significant difference, S: Significant, HS: Highly Significant

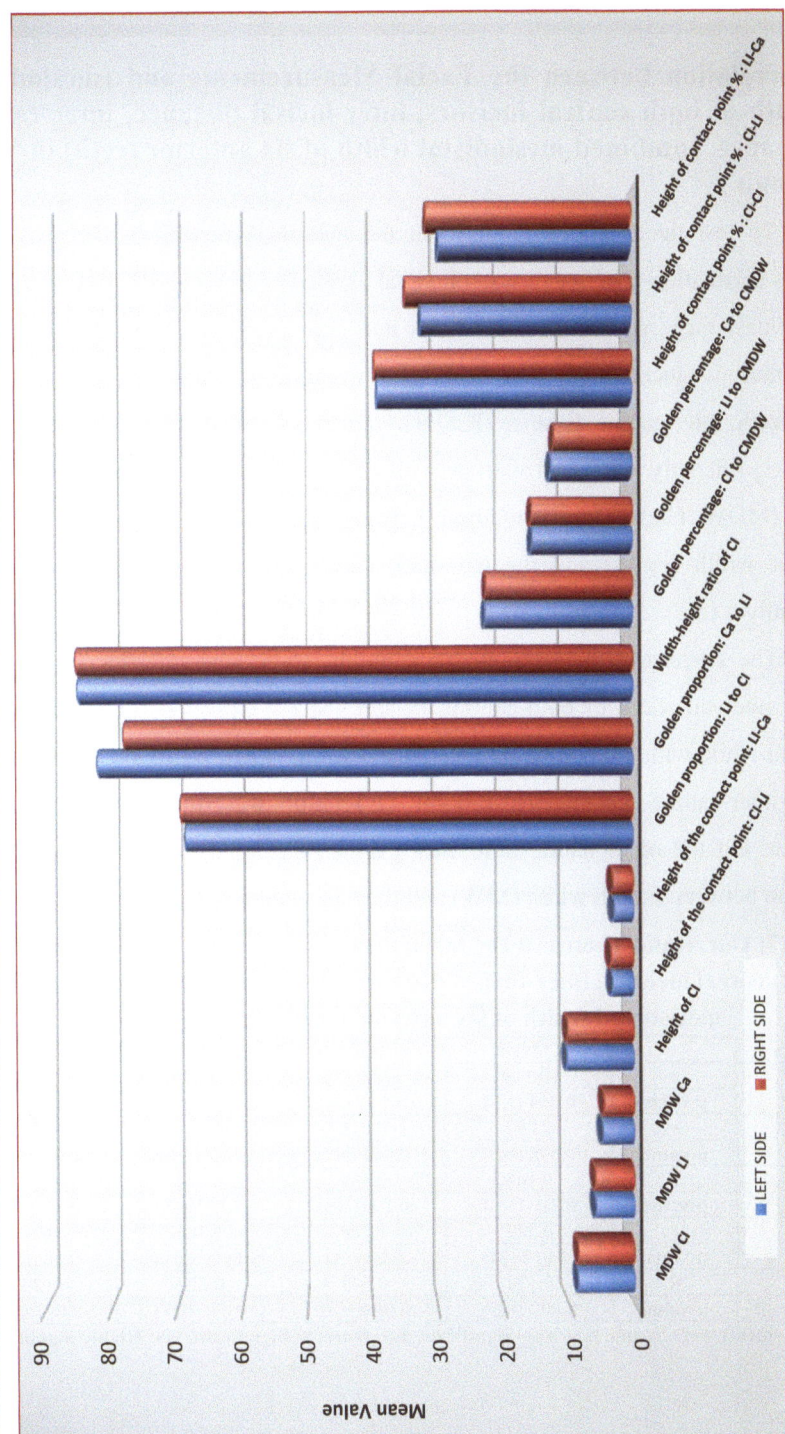

Figure 3.5: Descriptive statistics and side difference in micro-aesthetic appearance in female group.

3.7. Correlation between the Facial Measurements and (mesiodistal width of both central incisors, inter-incisal distance, inter-canine distance, combined mesiodistal width of six anterior teeth) in Male Group

To test the relationship between the measured variables in male group, Pearson's correlation coefficient was obtained as showed in table 3.7. According to r and p values, there was an indirect weak and non-significant correlation between inter-canthal distance (ICD) and combined mesiodistal width (CMDW) of six anterior teeth, inter-canine distance (ICaD) *and* inter-incisal distance (IID), and direct but non-significantly weak correlation with the mesiodistal width of both central incisors (MDW CIs). The correlation between the interpupillary width (IPW), zygomatic width (zy-zy) and the measured dental variables was direct and non-significantly weak.

The correlation between interalar width (IAW) and inter-incisal distance (IID), mesiodistal width of both central incisors (MDW CIS) was direct and highly significant while with the combined mesiodistal width (CMDW) of six anterior teeth and the inter-canine distance (ICaD) the correlation was direct and statistically significant. On the other hand, there was a direct and highly significant moderate correlation between mouth width (MW) and the measured dental variables.

Table 3.7: Correlation between the facial measurements and (mesiodistal width of both central incisors, inter-incisal distance, inter-canine distance, combined mesiodistal width of six anterior teeth) in male group.

Variables		CMDW	ICaD	IID	MDW CIs
ICD	r	-0.119	-0.070	-0.016	0.179
	p-value	0.364 (NS)	0.593(NS)	0.902 (NS)	0.172 (NS)
IPW	r	0.052	0.076	0.151	0.276
	p-value	0.696 (NS)	0.564 (NS)	0.250 (NS)	0.033 (NS)
zy-zy	r	0.164	0.169	0.204	0.210
	p-value	0.210 (NS)	0.196 (NS)	0.117(NS)	0.108 (NS)
IAW	r	0.329	0.280	0.360	0.377
	p-value	0.010 (S)	0.030 (S)	0.005 (HS)	0.003(HS)
MW	R	0.522	0.549	0.522	0.393
	p-value	0.000 (HS)	0.000(HS)	0.000 (HS)	0.002 (HS)

All measurements were in mm. NS: Non-Significant difference, S: Significant, HS: Highly Significant

3.8. Correlation between the Facial Measurements and (mesiodistal width of both central incisors, inter-incisal distance, inter-canine distance, combined mesiodistal width of six anterior teeth) in Female Group

To test the relationship between the measured variables in female group, Pearson's correlation coefficient was obtained as showed in table 3.8. According to r and p values, the correlation was weak, indirect and non-significant between the inter-canthal distance (ICD) and the measured dental variables, whereas the correlation between the interpupillary width (IPW) and combined mesiodistal width (CMDW) of six anterior teeth, mesiodistal width of both central incisors (MDW CIs) was direct and non-significantly weak and non-significantly weak and indirect correlation with inter-incisal distance (IID) and inter-canine distance (ICaD). On the other hand, there was a non-significantly weak and indirect correlation between the zygomatic width (zy-zy) and combined mesiodistal width (CMDW) of six anterior teeth, inter-incisal distance (IID), and a weak, direct and non-significant with the mesiodistal width of both central incisors (MDW CIs) and inter-canine distance (ICaD).

The correlation between the interalar width and combined mesiodistal width (CMDW) of six anterior teeth, inter-canine distance (ICaD) was weak, direct and non-significant and weak, indirect and non-significant with the inter-incisal distance (IID) and mesiodistal width of both central incisors (MDW CIs), while the correlation between the mouth width (MW) and the measured dental variables was weak, direct and statistically non-significant.

Table 3.8: Correlation the facial measurements and (mesiodistal width of both central incisors, inter-incisal distance, inter-canine distance, combined mesiodistal width of six anterior teeth) in female group.

Variables		CMDW	ICaD	IID	MDW CIs
ICD	r	-0.024	-0.052	-0.136	-0.097
	p-value	0.854 (NS)	0.692 (NS)	0.299 (NS)	0.460 (NS)
IPW	r	0.055	-0.009	-0.012	0.082
	p-value	0.678 (NS)	0.947 (NS)	0.928 (NS)	0.534 (NS)
zy-zy	r	-0.030	0.023	-0.117	0.095
	p-value	0.819 (NS)	0.863 (NS)	0.372 (NS)	0.471 (NS)
IAW	r	0.010	0.061	-0.104	-0.002
	p-value	0.940 (NS)	0.644 (NS)	0.431 (NS)	0.989 (NS)
MW	r	0.200	0.224	0.077	0.125
	p-value	0.126 (NS)	0.085 (NS)	0.558 (NS)	0.341 (NS)

All measurements were in mm. NS: Non-Significant difference, S: Significant, HS: Highly Significant

3.9. Correlation between Mesiodistal Width of each Tooth and the Facial Measurements in Male Group

Pearson's correlation coefficient for the measured variables in male group that demonstrated in table 3.9 indicated that there were:

A. A direct and highly significant correlation between:
- ✓ Interalar width (IAW) and mesiodistal width of left and right central incisors (MDW CI).
- ✓ Mouth width (MW) and mesiodistal width of left and right central (MDW CI) and lateral incisors (MDW LI) and left canine (MDW Ca).

B. A direct and significant correlation between:
- ✓ Interpupillary width (IPW) and mesiodistal width of right central incisor (MDW CI).

C. A direct and non-significant correlation between:
- ✓ Inter-canthal (ICD) distance and mesiodistal width of left and right central incisors (MDW CI).
- ✓ Interpupillary width (IPW) and mesiodistal width of left central incisor (MDW CI).

CHAPTER THREE

Results

- ✓ Zygomatic width (zy-zy) and mesiodistal width of left and right central (MDW CI) and lateral incisors (MDW LI) and mesiodistal width of left canine (MDW Ca).
- ✓ Interalar width (IAW) and mesiodistal width of left and right lateral incisors (MDW LI) and canines (MDW Ca).
- ✓ Mouth width (MW) and mesiodistal width of right canine (MDW Ca).
- ✓ Facial height (FH) and mesiodistal width of left and right central incisors (MDW CI) and left lateral incisor (MDW LI).
- ✓ Lower facial height (LFH) and mesiodistal width of left and right central incisors (MDW CI), left lateral incisor (MDW LI), left canine (MDW Ca).
- ✓ Upper lip vermilion (ULV) and mesiodistal width of left and right central incisors (MDW CI).
- ✓ Lower lip vermilion (LLV) and mesiodistal width of left and right central incisors (MDW CI), left lateral incisor (MDW LI), left canine (MDW Ca).

D. An indirect and non-significant correlation between:
- ✓ Inter-canthal distance (ICD) and mesiodistal width of left and right lateral incisors (MDW LI) and canines (MDW Ca).
- ✓ Interpupillary width (IPW) and mesiodistal width of left and right lateral incisors (MDW LI) and canines (MDW Ca).
- ✓ Zygomatic width (zy-zy) and mesiodistal of right canine (MDW Ca).
- ✓ Facial height (FH) and mesiodistal width of right and left canines (MDW Ca) and right lateral incisor (MDW LI).
- ✓ Lower facial height (LFH) and mesiodistal width of right lateral incisor and canine (MDW LI).
- ✓ Upper lip vermilion (ULV) and mesiodistal width of left and right lateral incisors (MDW LI) and canines (MDW Ca).
- ✓ Lower lip vermilion (LLV) and mesiodistal width of the right lateral incisor (MDW LI) and canine (MDW Ca).

Table 3.9: Correlation between mesiodistal width of each tooth and the facial measurements in male group.

Variables		MDW CI Left	MDW CI Right	MDW LI Left	MDW LI Right	MDW Ca Left	MDW Ca Right
ICD	R	0.185	0.160	-0.195	-0.196	-0.176	-0.187
	p-value	0.156 (NS)	0.222 (NS)	0.136 (NS)	0.134 (NS)	0.179 (NS)	0.153 (NS)
IPW	R	0.258	0.281	-0.099	-0.021	-0.042	-0.166
	p-value	0.046 (NS)	0.030 (S)	0.453 (NS)	0.876 (NS)	0.748 (NS)	0.205 (NS)
ZY-ZY	R	0.179	0.233	0.051	0.109	0.054	-0.016
	p-value	0.171 (NS)	0.073 (NS)	0.699 (NS)	0.409 (NS)	0.680 (NS)	0.902 (NS)
IAW	R	0.371	0.362	0.163	0.111	0.195	0.008
	p-value	0.004 (HS)	0.004 (HS)	0.214 (NS)	0.397 (NS)	0.136 (NS)	0.954 (NS)
MW	R	0.395	0.366	0.336	0.356	0.262	0.181
	p-value	0.002 (HS)	0.004 (HS)	0.009 (HS)	0.005 (HS)	0.043 (HS)	0.167 (NS)
FH	R	0.177	0.165	0.031	-0.047	-0.024	-0.206
	p-value	0.175 (NS)	0.206 (NS)	0.812 (NS)	0.722 (NS)	0.856 (NS)	0.115 (NS)
LFH	R	0.171	0.202	0.212	-0.057	0.084	-0.147
	p-value	0.191 (NS)	0.121 (NS)	0.104 (NS)	0.664 (NS)	0.526 (NS)	0.262 (NS)
ULV	R	0.091	0.155	-0.080	-0.055	-0.091	-0.257
	p-value	0.491 (NS)	0.237 (NS)	0.542 (NS)	0.678 (NS)	0.487 (NS)	0.047 (NS)
LLV	R	0.154	0.134	0.061	-0.116	0.042	-0.183
	p-value	0.240 (NS)	0.307 (NS)	0.644 (NS)	0.377 (NS)	0.749 (NS)	0.162 (NS)

All measurements were in mm. NS: Non-Significant difference, S: Significant, HS: Highly Significant

3.10. Correlation between the Mesiodistal Width of each Tooth and the Facial Measurements in Female Group

Pearson's correlation coefficient for the measured variables in female group that demonstrated in table 3.10 indicates that there were:

A. A direct and highly significant correlation between:
- ✓ Mouth width (MW) and mesiodistal width of left canine (MDW Ca).

B. A direct and non-significant correlation between:
- ✓ Inter-canthal distance (ICD) and mesiodistal width of left and right canines (MDW Ca).
- ✓ Interpupillary width (IPW) and mesiodistal width of left and right central incisors (MDW CI) and canines (MDW Ca).
- ✓ Zygomatic width (zy-zy) and mesiodistal width of left and right central incisors (MDW CI) and canines (MDW Ca).
- ✓ Interalar width (IAW) and mesiodistal width of left and right canines (MDW Ca) and left central incisor (MDW CI).

CHAPTER THREE   Results

- ✓ Mouth width (MW) and mesiodistal width of left and right central incisors (MDW CI), left lateral incisor (MDW LI) and right canine (MDW Ca).
- ✓ Facial height (FH) and mesiodistal width of left and right central incisors (MDW CI) and right canine (MDW Ca).
- ✓ Lower facial height (LFH) and mesiodistal width of the left and right central incisors (MDW CI) and canines (MDW Ca) and left lateral incisor (MDW LI).
- ✓ Upper lip vermilion (ULV) and mesiodistal width of left and right central (MDW CI) and lateral incisors (MDW LI) and right canine (MDW Ca).
- ✓ Lower lip vermilion (LLV) and mesiodistal width of left and right central (MDW CI) and lateral incisors (MDW LI) and left canine (MDW Ca).

C. An indirect and non-significant correlation between:
- ✓ Inter-canthal distance (ICD) and mesiodistal width of left and right central (MDW CIs) and lateral incisors (MDW LI).
- ✓ Interpupillary width (IPW) and mesiodistal width of left and right lateral incisors (MDW LI).
- ✓ Zygomatic width (zy-zy) and mesiodistal width of left and right lateral incisors (MDW LI).
- ✓ Interalar width (IAW) and mesiodistal width of left and right lateral incisors (MDW LI) and right central incisor (MDW CI).
- ✓ Mouth width (MW) and mesiodistal width of right lateral incisor (MDW LI).
- ✓ Facial height (FH) and mesiodistal width of left and right lateral incisors (MDW LI) and left canine (MDW Ca).
- ✓ Lower facial height (LFH) and mesiodistal width of right lateral incisor (MDW LI).
- ✓ Upper lip vermilion (ULV) and mesiodistal width of left canine (MDW Ca).
- ✓ Lower lip vermilion (LLV) and mesiodistal width of right canine (MDW Ca).

Table 3.10: Correlation between mesiodistal width of each tooth and the facial measurements in female group.

Variables		MDW CIs Left	MDW CIs Right	MDWLI Left	MDW LI Right	MDW Ca Left	MDW Ca Right
ICD	r	-0.065	-0.120	-0.123	-0.076	0.192	0.106
	p-value	0.622 (NS)	0.360 (NS)	0.349 (NS)	0.561 (NS)	0.142 (NS)	0.420 (NS)
IPW	R	0.117	0.046	-0.075	-0.103	0.083	0.146
	p-value	0.374 (NS)	0.728 (NS)	0.568 (NS)	0.431 (NS)	0.531 (NS)	0.267 (NS)
ZY-ZY	R	0.154	0.036	-0.252	-0.233	0.110	0.115
	p-value	0.239 (NS)	0.785 (NS)	0.052 (NS)	0.073 (NS)	0.402 (NS)	0.380 (NS)
IAW	R	0.013	-0.015	-0.115	-0.173	0.174	0.153
	p-value	0.919 (NS)	0.909 (NS)	0.380 (NS)	0.186 (NS)	0.183 (NS)	0.242 (NS)
MW	r	0.194	0.057	0.064	-0.089	0.361	0.121
	p-value	0.138 (NS)	0.667 (NS)	0.625 (NS)	0.498 (NS)	**0.005 (HS)**	0.358 (NS)
FH	r	0.127	0.015	-0.179	-0.177	-0.017	0.078
	p-value	0.332 (NS)	0.910 (NS)	0.172 (NS)	0.176 (NS)	0.900 (NS)	0.552 (NS)
LFH	r	0.219	0.185	0.012	-0.043	0.006	0.069
	p-value	0.093 (NS)	0.156 (NS)	0.927 (NS)	0.743 (NS)	0.963 (NS)	0.599 (NS)
ULV	r	0.198	0.236	0.136	0.098	-0.049	0.081
	p-value	0.129 (NS)	0.070 (NS)	0.299 (NS)	0.454 (NS)	0.711 (NS)	0.539 (NS)
LLV	R	0.173	0.169	0.209	0.070	0.048	-0.064
	p-value	0.186 (NS)	0.198 (NS)	0.109 (NS)	0.593 (NS)	0.717 (NS)	0.629 (NS)

All measurements were in mm. NS: Non-Significant difference, S: Significant, HS: Highly Significant

Chapter Four
Discussion

Enhancement of aesthetic appearance is one of the primary consideration for the patients that seeking orthodontic treatment, the term "appearance" is used in conjunction with the term "aesthetics" because it involves a broader assessment of the patient's face other than the teeth, so to achieve this goal, it is essential to make a comprehensive study of several facial and teeth factors to create a pleasing harmony of face and teeth **(Sarver, 2011; Jamayet *et al.*, 2014)**.

Orthodontists have been benefited from most of technological advancement in the diagnosis, orthodontic wires, and brackets, that result in more virtuous treatment times, this gives them more time for identifying micro-aesthetic characteristics and improving treatment outcomes to a degree that they have never been able to do before **(Sarver, 2011)**.

Two-dimensional photogrammetry has been used for evaluating and assessing the soft tissues and teeth in orthodontic treatment, this method was shown to be sufficiently non-invasive and reproducible, since it was simple to achieve in a conventional setting, without the need for a special equipment **(Edler *et al.*, 2003; Good *et al.*, 2006)**.

4.1. Sample

The sample in this study was selected at age between (18-23) years because the individuals maintain the same facial pattern till 25 years **(Bishara and Jakobsen, 1985)** and to minimize the effect of any remaining skeletal growth since the majority of facial growth is usually completed by the age of 16-17 years, as well as the occlusion at this age has been established regardless of the third molars **(Jones and Oliver, 2000)**.

| CHAPTER FOUR | Discussion |

4.2. Descriptive Statistics and Gender Differences in Macro-aesthetic Appearance

The human being faces have dimorphic features between genders, especially after puberty **(Kurkcuoglu *et al.*, 2013)**, and because males have longer growth period than females, the males were having larger measurements than females **(Subtenly, 1959; Trenouth *et al.*, 1985; Genecov *et al.*, 1990)**.

The differences in facial appearance between the males and females were clearly obvious in **table 3.2**. The mean values for facial parameters (macro-aesthetic appearance) were higher in males than females, this came in line with **Meredith and Chadha (1962); Marshall *et al.* (1986); Bishara *et al.* (1984, 1996); Ibrahimagić-Šeper *et al.* (2006); Ayoub *et al.* (2008); He *et al.* (2009); Ozdemir *et al.* (2009) and Dharap *et al.* (2013)**, since the lower mean values in facial parameters in females have been positively associated with improved facial beauty in females compared to males **(Raymond *et al.*, 2006)**.

One exception was found in upper and lower lip vermilion, the mean values for upper and lower lip vermilion were higher in females than males, this finding agreed with that of **Karaca *et al.* (2012); Asghari *et al.* (2014); Akinlolu *et al.* (2015)** and disagreed with that of **Ahmed *et al.* (2013); Kurkcuoglu *et al.* (2013)**, and could be attributed to that the aesthetically attractive female face demonstrated a larger lips, and this thought may be linked to the youthfulness and suggest a strong evolutionary effect on female attractiveness **(Peck and Peck, 1970; Foster, 1973; Peck and Peck, 1995)**.

4.3. Descriptive Statistics and Gender Differences in Maxillary Anterior Teeth Variables

The mean values for maxillary anterior teeth measurements for the right and the left sides were higher in males than in females, as shown in **table 3.3**, this agreed with **Al-Wazzan (1995); Al-Wazzan (2001); Ellakawa *et al.* (2011); Ahmed**

CHAPTER FOUR   Discussion

et al. **(2013); Shetty** *et al.* **(2013) and Sah** *et al.* **(2014),** and disagreed with **Murthy and Ramani (2008) and Jamayet** *et al.* **(2014)** which may be attributed to that the tooth size is determined to a large extent by genetic factors **(Horowitz** *et al.***, 1958; Lundetrom, 1964)**, so sex-linked inheritance was suggested **(Garn** *et al.***, 1965)**, since the differences between genders have a genetic basis that the possession of two X chromosomes in females provides a measure of control that lacked by males with only one X chromosome which lead to various developmental traits in the dentition of female including tooth size, but till now this hypothesis is not proved **(Garn** *et al.***, 1967)**.

    Additionally the height of left central incisor was significantly higher in males than in females; although the difference is statistically significant but it is too small in magnitude and may be clinically negligible. Also the mesiodistal width of both central incisors (MDW CIs), and inter-canine distance were significantly higher in males than in females, since the mesiodistal width of each central incisor was higher in males than females, while for the inter-canine distance, the males had a wider anterior teeth than females and this could be the reason behind the high significant gender difference in inter-canine distance.

    The finding regarding the central incisors supported by the results of **Ash (1984); Işcan and Kedici (2003)** in which the maxillary central incisors represent the most dominant anterior teeth as they can be seen in their full size and with their measurements, we can assess the racial and gender differences, since the males have a wider and longer anterior teeth in comparison to females **(Owens** *et al.***, 2002; Işcan and Kedici, 2003)**, but one exception was found regarding the measurements of the maxillary lateral incisor (right and left sides) which their mean values were higher in females than in males, this may be due to that the maxillary lateral incisor showed the greatest degree of variability in size than other teeth **(Lundstrom, 1948; Barrett** *et al.***, 1963; Lunt, 1969; Axelsson and Kirveskari, 1983; Murshid and Hashim, 1993).**

4.4 Descriptive Statistics and Gender Differences in Micro-aesthetic Appearance

There was a non-significant gender differences in micro-aesthetic appearance as shown in **table 3.4**, which agreed with **Fayyad *et al.* (2006); Nithya *et al.* (2008); Sulaiman *et al.* (2010); Umer *et al.* (2010); Chander *et al.* (2012); Forster *et al.* (2013) and Ahmed *et al.* (2014)**, and disagreed with **Parnia *et al.* (2010)**, this could be due to that the gender is not considered a significant factor and the proportions regarding the micro-aesthetic appearance were depending on the ethnic or racial characteristics rather than gender difference **((Fayyad *et al.*, 2006; Parnia *et al.*, 2010; Umer *et al.*, 2010)**.

Also, one exception was found regarding the golden proportion of the lateral incisor to central incisor (right side) which showed a significant gender difference, this finding came in accordance with **Parnia *et al.* (2010)**, and could be attributed to that the maxillary lateral incisor showed the greatest degree of variability in size than other teeth **(Lundstrom, 1948; Barrett *et al.*, 1963; Lunt, 1969; Axelsson and Kirveskari, 1983; proffit *et al.*, 1986; Murshid and Hashim, 1993)**.

The apperant proportions of the maxillary anterior teeth plays an important role in micro-aesthetics, the golden proportions were used as a yardstick to assess these proportions **(Naini *et al.*, 2006)**, in the present study, no existence of golden proportion in maxillary anterior teeth which supported the studies of **Preston (1993); Mahshid *et al.* (2004); Hasanreisoglu *et al.* (2005); Fayyad *et al.* (2006); Murthy and Ramani (2008); Chander *et al.* (2012); Naqash and Bali (2013); Azam *et al.* (2014) and Shah *et al.* (2014)**, and disagreed with **Levin (1973); Ward (2001); Pini *et al.* (2012)**, this may be attributed to the variations in the shape of maxillary arch **(Nikgoo *et al.*, 2009)** or to the alignment and positioning of anterior teeth **(Ong *et al.*, 2006)**, and as it was shown in **table 3.4**, the maxillary anterior tooth proportion was more than 66% for lateral to central incisor which was closer to the golden proportion than that of canine to lateral incisor which was more than 77%.

CHAPTER FOUR — Discussion

The maxillary central incisor considered the dominant tooth in the dental arch and the width /height ratio considered the most stable reference because it had a minimum variation among teeth **(Sah et al., 2014)**. In the present study, the ideal width/height ratio was 80% of the maxillary central incisor **(Gillen et al., 1994)** did not exist as shown in **table 3.4** and this was in accordance with **Garn et al. (1968); Lavelle (1972); Richardson (1975); Lennart and Nils (1982); McArthur (1985); Sterrett et al. (1999); Jullian and Rickne (2003); Magne et al. (2003); Hasanreisoglu et al. (2005); Wolfart et al. (2005); Singh (2006); Ku et al. (2012) and Sitthiphan et al. (2015)**, while disagreed with **Gillen et al. (1994); Marcushamer et al. (2011)**, this could be explained by the minor variation in dental traits among population types **(Bailit, 1975)**, the width/height ratio that was shown in **table 3.3** was more than 84%.

For the golden percentage for the maxillary anterior teeth, the results of the present study in **table 3.4** were differed from that suggested by Snow (10% for the canine, 15% for the lateral incisor, 25% for the central incisor of the total distance across the maxillary anterior segment), except for the lateral incisors which were very close to that suggested by Snow, this may be due to the curvature of the dental arch that could be the most critical factor in determining the golden percentage of maxillary anterior teeth **(Snow, 1999)**. This finding was consistent with **Fayyad et al. (2006); Murthy and Ramani (2008); Rita et al. (2013); Azam et al. (2014) and Calçada et al. (2014)**. The golden percentage for right and left sides as was shown in **table 3.4** were (more than 11% for canine, more than 15% and less than 16% for lateral incisor, *and* more than 22% for central incisor).

For the height of contact points between the maxillary anterior teeth, the results of the present study as shown in **table 3.4** were more than 38% for central incisor-central incisor, more than 33% for central incisor-lateral incisor, *and* more than 27% for lateral incisor-canine, this finding agreed with **Foulger et al. (2010); Stappert et al. (2010); Sghaireen et al. (2013) and Sghaireen et al. (2015);** and differed from the results of **Morley and Eubank (2001), Raj *et al*. (2009),** this could be attributed to the variation in the ethnicities of the populations.

4.5. Descriptive Statistics and Side Difference in Micro-aesthetic Appearance in Male and Female Group

Generally, as was shown in **table 3.5** for male group, there was a non-significant side difference in micro-aesthetic appearance which agreed with **Fayyad *et al*. (2006); Nithya *et al*. (2008); Forster *et al*. (2013); Rita *et al*. (2013) and Vadavadagi *et al*. (2015),** except in the height of contact point and height of contact point % between central incisor-lateral incisor *and* lateral incisor-canine, that showed a significant side difference; this could be attributed to that the lateral incisor showed a higher rate of asymmetry in comparison to other teeth **(Proffit *et al.*, 1986; Gallão *et al.*, 2009).**

On the other hand, **table 3.6** for female group showed in addition to the significant side difference in the height of contact point between central incisor-lateral incisor and height of contact point % between: central incisor-central incisor, central incisor-lateral incisor *and* lateral incisor- canine; it showed a high significant difference in mesiodistal width of canine, height of central incisor, golden proportion: canine to lateral incisor, golden percentage: canine to combined mesiodistal width (CMDW), this could be attributed to that the maxillary canines show the greatest degree of dimorphism **(Mavroskoufis and Ritchie, 1980; Nahidh, 2014; Orozco-Varo *et al.,* 2015),** and this came in line with **Gallão *et al*. (2009)** in that a slightly asymmetric maxillary lateral incisors and canines are usually very attractive because the more distant from the dental midline the lower is the demand for symmetry. Additionally, the unidentical dimensions of the right and left central incisors could be due to the fact "that two teeth can have identical dimensions when measured between certain reference points, but they may differ in outline form. This is because the portions of their outline form between the reference points may follow different curvatures" **(Mavroskoufis and Ritchie, 1980).**

4.6. Correlation between the Facial Measurements and (mesiodistal width of both central incisors, inter-incisal distance, inter-canine distance, combined mesiodistal width of six anterior teeth) in Male and Female Group

Generally, **table 3.7, 3.8** showed the relation between facial and dental measurements in male and female groups respectively. **In male group:** the **table 3.7** showed that the interpupillary width, zygomatic width, interalar and mouth width directly correlate with the maxillary anterior teeth variables which was in agreement with **Varjao and Nogueira (2006); Hussain *et al.* (2012); Mahesh *et al.* (2012); Sinavarat *et al.* (2013) and Strajnic *et al.* (2013),** and in disagreement with **Al Wazzan *et al.* (1995),** one exception was that the inter-canthal distance was indirectly correlate with combined mesiodistal width of maxillary anterior teeth, inter-canine distance and inter-incisal distance, this came in line with **Patel *et al.* (2011)** but disagreed with **Shah *et al.* (2015)** , statistically, the correlation was non-significant except in interalar and mouth width which had a statistically significant correlation with combined mesiodistal width of maxillary anterior teeth, inter-canine distance, inter-incisal distance, and mesiodistal width of both central incisors, which was consistent with **Al-El-Sheikh and Al-Athel (1998)**; **Hossain *et al.* (2012); Kini and Angadi (2012).**

In **female group:** the **table 3.8** showed that interpupillary width, zygomatic width, interalar and mouth width had a statistically non-significant and direct correlation with the measurements of maxillary anterior teeth, while a non-significant indirect correlation was found in the inter-canthal distance with the maxillary anterior teeth variables, interpupillary width with inter-canine distance and inter-incisal distance, zygomatic width with combined mesiodistal width of maxillary anterior teeth and inter-incisal distance *and* interalar width with inter-incisal distance,

CHAPTER FOUR

Discussion

and mesiodistal width of both central incisors, these finding agreed with **Patel *et al.* (2011)**; **Esan *et al.* (2012)**; **Sinavarat *et al.* (2013) and Strajnic *et al.* (2013)**; and disagreed with **Gomes *et al.* (2006); Hussain *et al.* (2012)**.

Regarding the correlation between (inter-canthal distance, interpupillary width, interalar, mouth width, zygomatic width) and (mesiodistal width of both central incisors, inter-incisal distance, inter-canine distance, combined Mesiodistal width of six anterior teeth), variation with other studies could be attributed to ethnic differences that exist between different populations, different instruments that used in studies and number of sample studied (**Hossain *et al.*, 2012; Hussain *et al,.* 2012; Kini and Angadi, 2012; Shah *et al.*, 2015**).

4.7. Correlation between Mesiodistal Width of each Tooth and the Facial Measurements in Male and Female Group

Table 3.9, 3.10 showed the correlation between mesiodistal width of each tooth and (inter-canthal, interpupillary, zygomatic width, interalar width, mouth width, facial height, lower facial height, upper lip vermilion, lower lip vermilion in male and female group respectively.

In male group, the table 3.9 showed the following:

-The inter-canthal distance had direct and statistically non-significant correlation with mesiodistal width of the left and right central incisor, this was in agreement with **Kassab (2005); Ariemba (2014)**, but had indirect correlation with mesiodistal width of the left and right lateral incisors and canines, this was in disagreement with **Al-Khatib *et al.* (2013)**.

-The interpupillary width had a non-significant direct correlation with mesiodistal width of left central incisor and significant direct correlation with mesiodistal width of right central incisor, this came in line with **Isa *et al.* (2010); Sharma *et al.* (2012),** and disagreed with **Al-Wazzan *et al.* (1995),** but had indirect and non-significant correlation with mesiodistal width of the left and right lateral incisors and canines.

CHAPTER FOUR

Discussion

-*The zygomatic width* had a statistically non-significant and direct correlation with mesiodistal width of the left and right central and lateral incisors and left canine, while it had a non-significant and indirect correlation with the mesiodistal width of right canine, this came in line with **Kassab (2005)**; **Sharma et al. (2012)**; **Jafari et al. (2014)** and disagree with **Al-Wazzan et al. (1995)**.

-*The interalar width* had a highly significant direct correlation with mesiodistal width of the left and right central incisors, and non-significant direct correlation with mesiodistal width of the left and right lateral incisors and canines, this disagreed with **Isa et al. (2010); Ariemba (2014)**.

-*The mouth width* had a highly significant direct correlation with mesiodistal width of the left and right central and lateral incisors, and left canine and non-significant direct correlation with mesiodistal width of the right canine, this consistent with **Kassab (2005); Al-Khatib et al. (2013)**, and in disagreement with **Al-Wazzan et al. (1995)**.

-*Facial height* had a non-significant direct correlation with mesiodistal width of the left and right central incisors and left lateral incisor *and* non-significant indirect correlation with mesiodistal width of the left and right canines and right lateral incisor; while *the lower facial height* had a non-significant direct correlation with mesiodistal width of the left and right central incisors, left lateral incisor and left canine, and non-significant indirect correlation with mesiodistal width of the right canine and right lateral incisor, this was in agreement with **Al-Khatib et al. (2013)** and disagree with **Ahmed et al. (2013)**.

-*The upper lip vermilion* had a non-significant direct correlation with mesiodistal width of the left and right central incisors, but had non-significant indirect correlation with mesiodistal width of the left and right lateral incisors and canines; while *the lower lip vermilion* had a non-significant indirect correlation with mesiodistal width of the right lateral incisor and canine, and has non-significant direct correlation with mesiodistal width of the left and right central incisors, left lateral incisor and canine, this was found to be in agreement with **Al-Khatib *et al.* (2013)**; **Ahmed *et al.* (2013)**.

In female group, the table 3.10 showed the following:

-The inter-canthal distance had a non-significant indirect correlation with mesiodistal width of the left and right central and lateral incisors, and non-significant direct correlation with mesiodistal width of the left and right canines, this came in line with **Ariemba (2014)**, and disagreed with **Kassab (2005)**.

-The interpupillary width had a non-significant direct correlation with mesiodistal width of the left and right central incisors and canines, and had a non-significant indirect correlation with mesiodistal width of the left and right lateral incisors, this came in line with **Kassab (2005); Ellakwa *et al.* (2011); Sharma *et al.* (2012)**, and disagreed with **Al-Wazzan *et al.* (1995)**.

-The zygomatic width had a non-significant direct correlation with mesiodistal width of the left and right central incisors and canines, and had a non-significant indirect correlation with mesiodistal width of the left and right lateral incisors, this came in line with **Kassab (2005); Jafari *et al.* (2014)**, and disagreed with **Sharma *et al.* (2012)**.

- The interalar width had a non-significant direct correlation with mesiodistal width of the left and right canines and left central incisor, and non-significant indirect correlation with mesiodistal width of the left and right lateral incisors and right central incisor, this was in agreement with **Al-Wazzan *et al.* (1995); Kassab (2005); Ellakwa *et al.* (2011); Ariemba (2014)**.

-The mouth width had highly significant direct correlation with mesiodistal width of the left canine, non-significant direct correlation with mesiodistal width of the left and right central incisors, left lateral incisor and right canine, and non-significant indirect correlation with mesiodistal width of the right lateral incisor, this was in agreement with **Kassab (2005); Al-Khatib *et al.* (2013)** and disagreed with **Al-Wazzan *et al.* (1995)**.

CHAPTER FOUR

Discussion

-*Facial height* had a non-significant direct correlation with mesiodistal width of the left and right central incisors and right canine, this came in line with **Al-Khatib et al. (2013)** *and* non-significant indirect correlation with mesiodistal width of the left and right lateral incisors and left canines, this was in agreement with **Ahmed et al. (2013)**; while *the lower facial height* had a non-significant direct correlation with mesiodistal width of the left and right central incisors, canines and left lateral incisor, and non-significant indirect correlation with mesiodistal width of the right lateral incisor, this was consistent with **Al-Khatib et al. (2013)**.

-**The upper lip vermilion** had a non-significant direct correlation with mesiodistal width of the left and right central and lateral incisors and right canine, this was in agreement with **Al-Khatib et al. (2013)**, but had non-significant indirect correlation with mesiodistal width of the left canine which came in line with **Ahmed et al. (2013)**; while *the lower lip vermilion* had non-significant indirect correlation with mesiodistal width of the right canine, *and* non-significant direct correlation with mesiodistal width of the left and right central and lateral incisors, left canine, this found to be in agreement with **Al-Khatib et al. (2013)**.

The variations regarding correlation between mesiodistal width of each tooth and (inter-canthal, interpupillary, zygomatic width, interalar width, mouth width, facial height, lower facial height, upper lip vermilion, lower lip vermilion) in male and female group in different studies could be attributed to the differences in the ethnicities of the populations studied, in measuring techniques and number of samples studied (**Hossain et al., 2012; Hussain et al,. 2012; Kini and Angadi, 2012; Shah et al., 2015**).

4.8 Clinical Consideration

In the past, the cephalometric analysis represented an important tool in orthodontic treatment planning, but today, the focus is mainly on facial soft tissue and dental assessment by using photographs. Despite that most of orthodontists focused primarily on occlusal desicrepancies and mal-relations when discussed the needs of

CHAPTER FOUR

Discussion

treatment with the patients, and the patients and parents focused mainly on appearance, the orthodontic diagnosis and treatment planning should has a broader scope, include the occlusion, tooth shape and appearance of the face to have both excellent occlusion and excellent aesthetics, although this is quite difficult but it is the goal that all orthodontists should pursue to.

Although orthodontists do not perform the dental procedures that related to cosmetics such as composite bonding, but there are principles in cosmetic dentistry that orthodontists can use to enhance the aesthetic outcomes of the finished cases. One of the most important issues in orthodontics is how to gain space (for example: by interproximal reduction) or get rid of excess space (for example: by composite bonding or veneers), additionally, existance of tooth size discrepancy (TSD) which means disproportion or lack of harmony of mesiodistal dimension of teeth when related to those within the same arch or the opposing arch, represents one of the major problems in orthodontics, these problems could be overcomed by considering anterior teeth dimensions and proportions, the present study describe the normative values of micro-aesthetic appearance "dental proportions and dimensions" and their relation to facial measurements in a sample of Iraqi population, which should be considered by the orthodontists for treatment finishing.

Although the concerns and actions of orthodontists are measured in millimeters, they can improve and make a difference in patient's life, therefore; the micro-aesthetics should not be seen in isolation but, as a key to provide a pleasant smile "mini-aesthetics" and harmonious face "macro-aesthetics".

Additionally, the differences in dental measurements and in the right and left sides in male and female groups could be beneficial in forensic dentistry by comparison of tooth dimensions in males and females by using ante-mortem (prior to death) and post-mortem (after death) photographs to identify the person to whom the teeth belong, since the teeth provide resistance to damage in terms of fire and bacterial decomposition when the rest of body is damaged.

Chapter Five
Conclusions and suggestions

5.1. Conclusions

A. Photographical analysis of macro-aesthetic appearance in both genders:
* Most of the mean values of macro-aesthetic appearance were significantly higher in males than females, so that gender differences exist in facial measurements.

B. Photographical analysis of micro-aesthetic appearance and side difference in both genders:
* The micro-aesthetic appearance measurements were mostly higher in females than males, since the gender has no effect on maxillary anterior teeth proportions.
* No existence of golden proportion in maxillary anterior teeth with maxillary lateral to central incisors proportions were closer to that of golden proportion.
* No existence of normal width/height ratio of maxillary central incisors, and the maxillary central incisors were wider than normal.
* The maxillary lateral incisors were the only teeth that have a golden percentage very close to the golden percentage, whereas the golden ratio did not exist in the height of contact point between the maxillary anterior teeth.
* The maxillary lateral incisor showed a significant side difference in male and female group, whereas the maxillary canine showed a significant side difference in female group only.

C. The relationship between facial and dental measurements:
* Generally, there was a non-significant correlation between most of the facial and maxillary anterior teeth measurements in both genders.

References

- **Abdulhadi L, Mohammed H.** Mathematic method to calculate the central incisor form using face records and vice versa. J Bio and Biomed Eng 2012; 6(1): 9-14.
- **Adamson PA, Zavod MB.** Changing perceptions of beauty: a surgeon's perspective. Facial Plast Surg 2006; 22(3): 188-193.
- **Adolfi D.** Functional, esthetic, and morphologic adjustment procedures for anterior teeth. Quintessence Dent Technol 2009; 32: 153-168.
- **Ahmad I.** Anterior dental aesthetics: historical perspective. Br Dent J 2005; 198(12): 737-742.
- **Ahmed HM, Al-labban Y, Nahidh M.** Facial measurements and maxillary anterior teeth mesiodistal dimensions, is there a relationship?. Iraqi Dent J 2013; 35(2): 39-43.
- **Ahmed N, Abbas M, Maqsood A.** Evaluation of recurring esthetic dental proportion innatural smile of Pakistani sample. Pakistan Oral & Dental Journal 2014; 34(4): 739-742.
- **Akinlolu AA, Akinola BO, Nurudeen RL, Kadiri RE, Ajao MS.** Cephalometric study of mouth morphology among major nigerian tribes. Anatomy Journal of Africa 2015; 4(1): 496-504.
- **Aksakalli S, Demir A.** The comparison of facial estethics between orthodontically treated patients and their parents. The Scientific World Journal 2013; 3: 903507.
- **Al-El-Sheikh HM, Al-Athel MS.** The relationship of interalar width, interpupillary width and maxillary anterior teeth width in Saudi population. Odontostomatol Trop 1998; 21(84): 7-10.
- **Al-Johany SS, Alqahtani AS, Alqahtani FY, Alzahrani AH.** Evaluation of different esthetic smile criteria. Int J Prosthodont 2011; 24(1): 64-70.

References

- **Al-Khatib AR, Rajion ZA, Masudi SM, Hassan R, Townsend GC.** Dento-facial relationships in individuals with normal occlusion. HOMO-Comparative Human Biology J 2013; 64(4): 296-311.
- **Alley TF, Cunningham MR.** Averaged faces are attractive, but very attractive faces are not average. Psychological Science 1991; 2(2): 123-125.
- **Al-Marzok M, Majeed K, Ibrahim I.** Evaluation of maxillary anterior teeth and their relation to the golden proportion in Malaysian population. BMC Oral Health 2013; 13(1): 9.
- **Al-Ramahi SCA.** Evaluation of buccal corridor in posed smile for Iraqi adults sample with class I normal occlusion. A master thesis, Department of Orthodontics, University of Baghdad, 2009.
- **Al-Sehaibany F.** Analysis of maxillary anterior teeth and various facial dimensions among adolescents in riyadh, saudi Arabia. JPDA 2011; 20(2): 67-72.
- **Al-Wazzan K, Al Haidan A, Al Madi E, Al Mufarj A.** The relationship between facial references and mesiodistal width of maxillary anterior teeth among Saudi patients. Adj 1995; 20(4): 39-45.
- **Al-Wazzan KH.** The relationship between intercanthal dimension and the widths of maxillary anterior teeth. J Prosthet Dent 2001; 86(6): 608-612.
- **Al-Zubaydi FS.** Evaluation of the gingival smile line in class I pattern in Iraqi sample aged 18-25: a comparative clinical and cephalometric study. A Master Thesis, Department of Orthodontics, Collage of Dentistry, University of Baghdad, 2005.
- **Andrews LF.** The six keys to normal occlusion. Am J Orthod 1972; 62(3): 296-309.
- **Andrews LF.** Straight wire: the concept and appliance. San Diego, CA: LA Wells, 1989.
- **Angle EH.** Classification of malocclusion. Dent Cosmos 1899; 41(3): 248-264.

References

- **Ariemba Rm.** Relationship between the nasal, inner-canthal and mesiodistal widths of the maxillary anterior teeth in a Kenyan population. Master Thesis. Department of Conservative and Prosthetic Dentistry, School of Dental Sciences, University of Nairobi, 2014.
- **Aristoteles.** The Works of Aristotle-volume IV: historia animalium. Oxford: clarendon press. 1949, cited by Vegter F, Hage JJ. Clinical anthropometry and canons of the face in historical perspective. Plast Reconstr Surg 2000; 106(5): 1090-1096.
- **Aristotle.** Nicomachean ethics. 1094a, cited by Prokopakis EP, Vlastos IM, Picavet V, Trenité GN, Thomas R, Cingi C, Hellings PW. The golden ratio in facial symmetry. Rhinology 2013; 51(1): 18-21.
- **Asghari A, Rajaeih S, Hassannia F, Tavakolifard N, Neisyani HF, Kamrava SK, Jalessi M, Omidian P.** Photographic facial soft tissue analysis of healthy Iranian young adults: anthropometric and angular measurements. Med J Islam Repub Iran 2014; 28:49.
- **Ash MM.** Wheeler's atlas of tooth form. 5th ed, Philadelphia: Saunders, 1984.
- **Axelsson G, Kirveskari P.** Crown size of permanent teeth in Icelanders. Acta Odont Scand 1983; 41(3): 181-186.
- **Ayoub F, Yehia M, Rizk A, Al-Tannir M, Abi- Farah A, Hamadeh G.** Forensic norms of female and male Lebanese adults. J Forensic Odontol stomatol 2008; 27(1): 18-23.
- **Azam S, Shahnawaz A, Qureshi B.** Validity of esthetic proportions in maxillary anterior teeth. POJ 2014; 6(1): 7-11.

B

- **Baig MA.** Surgical enhancement of facial beauty and its psychological significance. Annals of the Royal Australasian College of Dental Surgeons 2004; 17: 64-67.

References

- **Bailit HL**. Dental variations among populations: an anthropologic view. Dent Clin North Am 1975; 19(1): 125-139.
- **Baldwin DC**. Appearance and aesthetics in oral health. Community Dent Oral Epidemiol 1980; 8: 224-256.
- **Barker DJ, Barker MJ**. The body as art. Journal of Cosmetic Dermatology 2002; 1(2): 88-93
- **Barrett MJ, Brown T, MacDonald MR**. Dental observations on Australian aborigines: mesiodistal crown diameters of permanent teeth. Aust Dent J 1963; 8(2): 150-155.
- **Bashour M**. An objective system for measuring facial attractiveness. Plast Reconstr Surg 2006; 118(3): 757-776.
- **Baume LJ, Horowitz HS, Summers CJ, Backer Dirkes O, Carlos JP, Cohn LK**. A method for measuring occlusal traits developed by FDI commission on classification and statistics for oral conditions. Int Dent J 1973; 23(3): 530-537.
- **Baumrind S, Frantz RC**. The reliability of head film measurements 1. landmark identification. Am J Orthod 1971; 60(2): 111-127.
- **Behrents R**. "JCO/interviews Dr. Rolf Behrents on adult craniofacial growth". Journal of Clinical Orthodontics 1986; 20(12): 842-847.
- **Bell WH, Jacobs JD, Quejada JG**. Simultaneous repositioning of the maxilla, mandible and chin. Am J Orthod 1986; 89(1): 28-50.
- **Benson PE, Richmond S**. A critical appraisal of measurement of the soft tissue out line using photographs and video. Eur J orthod 1997; 19(4): 397-409.
- **Bishara SE**. Text book of orthodontics. Saunders, Philadelphia, 2001.
- **Bishara SE, Peterson L, Bishara EC**. Changes in facial dimensions and relationships between the ages of 5 and 25 years. Am J Orthod 1984; 85(3): 238-252.
- **Bishara SE, Jakobsen JR, Jorgensen GJ**. Changes in facial dimensions. Am J Orthod Dentofac Orthop 1995; 108(4): 389-393.

References

- **Bishara SE, Jacobsen JR, Angelakis D**. Post-treatment changes in male and female patients: a comparative study. Am J Ortho Dentofac Orthop 1996; 110(6): 624-629.
- **Bjork A**. Facial growth in man, studied with the aid of metallic implants. Acta Odontol Scand 1955; 13(1): 9-34.
- **Bolton WA**. The clinical application of a tooth-size analysis. Am J Orthod 1962; 48: 504-529.
- **Brandão RCB, Brandão LBC**. Finishing procedures in orthodontics: dental dimensions and proportions (microesthetics). Dental Press J Orthod 2013; 18(5): 147-174.
- **British Standard Institution**. Glossary of dental term (BS4492). London: BSI. 1983, cited by: Jones ML, Oliver RG. W&H orthodontic notes. 6th ed. Oxford: Wright, 2000: 62.
- **Broadbent BH**. A new X-ray technique and its application to orthodontia. Angle Orthod 1931; 1(2): 45-66.
- **Burke PH, Beard FH**. Stereophotogrammetry of the face. A preliminary investigation into the accuracy of a simplified system evolved for contour mapping by photography. Am J Orthod 1967; 53(10): 769-782.
- **Burstone C**. Integumental contour and extension patterns. Angle Orthod 1959; 29(2): 93-104.

C

- **Calçada D, Correia A, Araújo F**. Anthropometric analysis of anterior maxillary teeth with digital photography-a study in a Portuguese sample. Int J Esthet Dent 2014; 9(3): 370-380.
- **Câmara CA**. Aesthetics in orthodontics: six horizontal smile lines. Dental Press J 2010; 15(1): 118-131.
- **Cassin B, Solomon S**. Dictionary of eye terminology. Gainsville, Florida: Triad Publishing Company, 1990.

References

- **Cesario VA, Latta GH**. Relationship between the mesiodistal width of the maxillary central incisor and interpupillary distance. J Prosthet Dent 1984; 52(5): 641-643.
- **Chander NG, Kumar VV, Rangarajan V**. Golden proportion assessment between maxillary and mandibular teeth on Indian population. J Adv Prosthodont 2012; 4(2): 72-75.
- **Chang ZC, Hu FC, Lai E, Yao CC, Chen MH, Chen YJ**. Landmark identification errors on cone-beam computed tomography-derived cephalograms and conventional digital cephalograms. Am J Orthod Dentofac Orthop 2011; 140(6): 289-297.
- **Chu M**. The accuracy of photogrammetric measurements employed in the analysis of facial morphology. Master Thesis. 1989, cited by Payne MG. The reliability of facial soft tissue landmarks with photogrammetry. Master's Thesis, Marquette University, 2013.
- **Claman LC, Patton D, Rashid R**. Standardized portrait photography for dental patient. Am J Orthod Dentofac Orthop 1990; 98(3): 197-205.
- **Claus EB, Calvocoressi L, Bondy ML, Schildkraut JM, Wiemels JL, Wrensch M**. Dental x-rays and risk of meningioma. Cancer 2012; 118(18): 4530-4537.
- **Clifford M, Walster E**. The effects of physical attractiveness on teacher expectation. Sociol Educ 1973; 46(2): 248-258.
- **Collins M**. The eye of the beholder: face recognition and perception. Semin Orthod 2012; 18: 229-234.
- **Cooke MS, Stephen HY**. The reproducibility of natural head posture: a methodological study. Am J Orthod Dentofac Orthop 1988; 93(4): 280-288.
- **Cooper GE, Tredwin CJ, Cooper NT**, Petrie A, Gill DS. The influence of maxillary central incisor height-to-width ratio on perceived smile aesthetics. Br Dent J 2012; 212(12): 589-599.

References

- **Costa JR, Prates JC, De Castilho HT, Santos RA**. Estudiocraneométrico de los huesosnasalesyproceso frontal de la maxila. Int J Morphol 2005; 23(1): 9-12, cited by Al-Janabi SM. Photogrammetric analysis of facial soft tissue profile of Iraqi adults sample with class I normal occlusion. A master thesis, Department of Orthodontics, University of Baghdad, 2011.
- **Cunningham SJ**. The psychology of facial appearance. Dent Update 1999; 26(10): 438-443.

D

- **DeBruine LM, Jones BC, Unger L, Little AC, Feinberg DR**. Dissociating averageness and attractiveness: attractive faces are not always average. J ExpPsychol Hum Percept Perform 2007; 33(6): 1420-1430.
- **Dharap A, Salem A, Fadel R, Osman M, Chakravarty M, Abdul Latif N, Abu-Hijleh M**. Facial anthropometry in an Arab population. Bahrain Med Bull 2013; 35(2): 60-65.
- **Dickason WL, Hanna D**. Pitfalls of comparative photography in plastic and reconstructive surgery. Am J Orthod 1976; 58(11): 166-175.
- **Draker HL**. Hand capping labio-lingual deviations: a proposed index for public health purposes. Am J Orthod 1960; 46(4): 295-305.

E

- **Edler RJ**. Background considerations to facial aesthetics. J Orthod 2001; 28(2): 159-168.
- **Edler R, Wertheim D, Greenhill D**. Comparison of radiographic and photographic measurement of mandibular asymmetry. Am J Orthod Dentofac Orthop 2003; 123(2): 167-174.
- **Ellakwa A, McNamara K, Sandhu J, James K, Arora A, Klineberg I, El-Sheikh A, Martin FE**. Quantifying the selection of maxillary anterior teeth using

intraoral and extraoral anatomical landmarks. J Contemp Dent Pract 2011; 12(6): 414-421.
- **Esan TA, Oziegbe OE, Onapokya HO**. Facial approximation: evaluation of dental and facial proportions with height. African Health Sciences 2012; 12(1): 63-68.
- **Etezad-Razavi M, Jalalifar S**. Correlation between interpupillary and inner-outer intercanthal distances in individuals younger than 20. J Ophthalmic Vis Res, 2008; 3(1): 16-22.
- **Evison M, Dryden I, Fieller N, Mallett X, Morecroft L, Schofield D, Bruegge RV**. Key parameters of face shape variation in 3D in a large sample. J Forensic Sci 2010; 55(1): 159-162.

F

- **Farias F, Ennes J, Zorzatto R**. Aesthetic value of the relationship between the shapes of the face and permanent upper central incisor. Inter J of Dent 2010: 6.
- **Farkas LG**. Results. In: Farkas, LG and Munro, IR (Eds.), Anthropometric facial proportions in medicine. Springfield, III: Charles C Thomas, 1987; 155-319.
- **Farkas LG**. Examination. In: Farkas LG (Ed). Anthropometry of the head and face, 2nd Ed. New York: Raven Press, 1994; 20-26.
- **Farkas LG, Ross RB, James JS**. Anthropometry of the face in lateral dysplasia: the bilateral form. Cleft Palate J 1977; 14(1): 41-51.
- **Farkas LG, Hajnis K, Posnick JC**. Anthropometric and anthroposcopic findings of the nasal and facial region in cleft patients before and after primary lip and palate repair. Cleft Palate Craniofac J 1993; 30(1): 1-12.
- **Farkas LG, Katic MJ, Forrest CR, Alt KW, Bagic I, Baltadjiev G, et al,**. International anthropometric study of facial morphology in various ethnic groups/races. J Cranio fac Surg 2005; 16(4): 615-646.
- **Faure JC, Rieffe C, Maltha JC**. The influence of different facial components on facial aesthetics. Eur J Orthod 2002; 24(1): 1-7.

References

- **Fayyad MA, Jamani KD, Aqrabawi J**. Geometric and mathematical proportions and their relations to maxillary anterior teeth. J Contemp Dent Pract 2006; 7(5): 62-70.
- **Fazel R, Krumholz HM, Wang Y, Ross JC, Chen J, Ting HH, et al,**. Exposure to low-dose ionizing radiation from medical imaging procedures. N Engl J Med 2009; 361(9): 849-857.
- **Fernández-Riveiro P, Smyth-Chamosa E, Suárez-Quintanilla D, Suárez-Cunqueiro M**. Angular photogrammetric analysis of the soft tissue facial profile. Eur J Orthod 2003; 25(3): 393-399.
- **Ferrario VF, Sforza C, Schmitz JH, Ciusa V, Colombo A**. Normal growth and development of the lips: a 3-dimensional study from 6 years to adulthood using a geometric model. J Anat 2000; 196(3): 415-423.
- **Fink B, Neave N, Manning JT, Grammer K**. Facial symmetry and judgements of attractiveness, health and personality. Personality and Individual Differences 2006; 41(3): 491-499.
- **Finlay F**. Craniometry and cephalometry: a history prior to the advent of radiography. Angle Orthod 1980; 50(4): 312-321.
- **Formby WA, Nanda RS, Currier GF**. Longitudinal changes in the adult facial profile. Am J Orthod Dentofac Orthop 1994; 105(5): 464-476.
- **Forster A, Velez R, Antal M, Nagy K**. Width ratios in the anterior maxillary region in a Hungarian population: addition to the golden proportion debate. J Prosthet Dent 2013; 110(3): 211-215.
- **Foster EJ**. Profile preferences among diversified groups. Angle Orthod 1973; 43(1): 34-40.
- **Foster TD**. A text book of orthodontics. 2nd ed. Oxford: Blackwell Scientific Publication, 1985: 14, 34-36.

References

- **Foulger TE, Tredwin CJ, Gill DS, Moles DR**. The influence of varying maxillary incisal edge embrasure space and interproximal contact area dimensions on perceived smile aesthetics. Br Dent J 2010; 209(3): 4.
- **Fourie Z, Damstra J, Gerrits PO, Ren Y**. Evaluation of anthropometric accuracy and reliability using different three-dimensional scanning systems. Forensic Science International 2011; 207(1): 127-134.
- **Frankel R, Frankel C**. Orthodontics in orofacial region with help of function regulators. Inf Orthod Kieferorthop 1988; 20: 277-309.

G

- **Gallão S, Ortolani C, Santos-Pinto A, Santos-Pinto L, Junior K**. Photographic analysis of symmetry and aesthetic proportion of the anterior teeth. Rev Inst Ciênc Saúde 2009; 27(4): 400-404.
- **Garn SM, Lewis AB, Kerewsky RS**. X-linked inheritance of tooth size. J Dent Res 1965; 44(2): 439-441.
- **Garn SM, Lewis AB, Swindler DR. Kerewsky RS**. Genetic control of sexual dimorphism in tooth size. J Dent Res 1967; 46(2): 963-972.
- **Gavan JA, Washburn SL, Lewis PH**. Photography: An anthropometric tool. Am J Phys Anthrop 1952; 10(3): 331-351.
- **Genecov JS, Sinclair PM, Dechow PC**. Development of the nose and soft tissue profile. Angle Orthod 1990; 60(3): 191-198.
- **Ghoddousi H, Edler R, Haers P, Wertheim D, Greenhill D**. Comparison of three methods of facial measurement. Int J Oral Maxillofac Surg 2007; 36(3): 250-258.
- **Gillen RJ, Schwartz RS, Hilton TJ, Evans DB**. An analysis of selected normative tooth proportions. Int J Prosthodont 1994; 7(5): 410-417.
- **Gomes Vl, Gonçalves Lc, Costa Mm, lucas Bd**. Interalar distance to estimate the combined width of the six maxillary anterior teeth in oral rehabilitation treatment. J Esthet Restor Dent 2009; 21(1): 26-36.

References

- **Gomes Vl, Gonçalves Lc, Prado C, Junior I, Lucas B**. Correlation between facial measurements and the mesiodistal width of the maxillary anterior teeth. J Esthet Restor Dent 2006; 18(4): 196-205.
- **Good S, Edler R, Wertheim D, Greenhill D**. A computerized photographic assessment of the relationship between skeletal discrepancy and mandibular outline asymmetry. Eur J Orthod 2006; 28(2): 97-102.
- **Gordon P, Wander P**. Technique for dental photography. J Clin Orthod 1987; 21(2): 362-370.
- **Gosman SD**. Anthropometric method of facial analysis in orthodontics. Am J Orthod 1950; 36(10): 749-762.
- **Graber TM, Vanarsdall RL**. A text book of orthodontics, current principles and techniques, 3rd ed. Mosby, Inc, 2000: 14-16.
- **Graber TM, Vanarsdall RL, Vig KW, Xubair A**. A text book of orthodontics, current principles and techniques, 5th ed. Mosby, Inc, 2012.
- **Gribel BF, Gribel MN, Frazao DC, McNamara JA, Manzi FR**. Accuracy and reliability of craniometric measurements on lateral cephalometry and 3D measurements on CBCT scans. Angle Orthod 2011; 81(1): 26-35.
- **Gurel G**. The science and art of porcelain laminate veneers. New Malden, Surrey, United Kingdom, London: Quintessence, 2003: 83-86.

H

- **Hajeer MY, Millett DT, Ayoub AF, Siebert JP**. Applications of 3D imaging in orthodontics: part I. J Orthod 2004; 31(1): 62-70.
- **Haraguchia S, Iguchib Y, Takadac K**. Asymmetry of the face in orthodontic patients. Angle Orthod 2008; 78(3): 421-426.
- **Hasanreisoglu U, Berksun S, Aras K, Arsalan I**. An analysis of maxillary anterior teeth: facial and dental proportions. J Prosthet Dent 2005; 94(6): 530-538.

References

- **He Z, Jian X, Wu X, Gao X, Zhou S, Zhong X**. Anthropometric measurement and analysis of the external nasal soft tissue in 119 young Han Chinese adults. J Craniofac Surg 2009; 20(5): 1347-1351.
- **Heinemann W**. Aristotle-minor works: physiognomics. Cambridge, Mass.: Harvard University Press, 1963: 83-137.
- **Hellman M**. Some facial features and their orthodontic implication. Am J Orthod Oral Surg 1939; 25(10): 927-951.
- **Hilhorst MT**. Physical beauty: only skin deep?. Medicine, Health Care and Philosophy 2002; 5(1): 11-21.
- **Holdaway RA**. A soft-tissue cephalometric analysis and its use in orthodontic treatment planning. Part-I. Am J Orthod Dentofac Orthop 1983; 84: 1-28.
- **Horowitz SL, Osborne RH, DeGeorge FV**. Hereditary factors in tooth dimensions: A study of the anterior teeth of twins. Angle Orthod 1958; 28(2): 87-93.
- **Hosoda M, Stone-Romero EF, Coats G**. The effects of physical attractiveness on job-related outcomes: a meta-analysis of experimental studies. Personnel Psychol 2003; 56(2): 431-462.
- **Hossain S, Islam KZ, Islam KMM**. Correlation between maxillary canines and facial anatomical landmarks in a group of Bangladeshi people. City Dental College J 2012; 9(2): 12-14.
- **Houston WJB, Stephens CD, Tulley WJ**. A Textbook of orthodontics. Great Britain: Wright 1992: 1-13.
- **Howells DJ, Shaw WC**. The validity of rating of dental and facial attractiveness for epidemiologic use. Am J Orthod 1985; 88(5): 400-408.
- **Hrdlicka A**. Practical anthropometry. Philadelphia: Wistar Institute of Anatomy and Biology, 1920.

References

- **Hunt O, Hepper P, Johnston C, Stevenson M, Burden D**. The aesthetic component of the index of orthodontic treatment need validated against lay opinion. Eur J Orthod 2002; 24(1): 53-59.
- **Huntley HE**. The divine proportion: a study in mathematical beauty. New York: Dover, 1970.
- **Hussain Mw, Qamar K, Naeem S**. The role of interpupillary distance in the selection of anterior teeth. Pakistan Oral & Dental Journal 2012; 32(1): 165-169.

I

- **Işcan MY, Kedici PS**. Sexual variation in bucco-lingual dimensions in Turkish dentition. Forensic Sci Int 2003; 137(2-3): 160-164.
- **Ibrahimagić- Šeper L, Čelebić A, Petričević N, Selimović E**. Anthropometric differences between males and females in face dimensions and dimensions of central maxillary incisors. Medicinski glasnik 2006; 3(2): 58-62.
- **Iliffe AH**. A study of preferences in feminine beauty. British Journal of Psychology 1960; 51(3): 267-273.
- **Isa ZM, Tawfiq OF, Noor NM, Shamsudheen MI, Rijal MO**. Regression methods to investigate the relationship between facial measurements and widths of the maxillary anterior teeth. J Prosthet Dent 2010; 103(3): 182-188.

J

- **Jabir S**. Facial beauty-a primer on its determinants. PSJT 2014; 1(4): 26-30.
- **Jafari H, Radmehr O, Kaviani R, Valaei N**. The analysis of correlation between the facial width and mesiodistal width of the maxillary anterior teeth. J Res Dent Sci 2014; 11(1): 49-53.
- **Jamayet NB, Viwattanatipa N, Amornvit P, Pornprasertsuk S, Jira Chindasombatjaroen J, Alam MK**. Comparison of crown width/length ratio of six maxillary anterior teeth between different facial groups in Bangladeshi population. IMJ 2014; 21(1): 49-54.

References

- **Jefferson Y.** Facial beauty-establishing a universal standard. IJO 2004; 15(1): 9-22.
- **Jones ML, Oliver RG.** W&H orthodontic notes. 6th ed. Oxford: Wright. 2000: 1-2, 24, cited by Al-Ramahi SCA. Evaluation of buccal corridor in posed smile for Iraqi adults sample with class I normal occlusion. A master thesis, Department of Orthodontics, University of Baghdad, 2009.

K

- **Karaca Ö, Gülcen B, Kuş MA, Elmali F, Kuş İ.** Morphometric facial analysis of Turkish adults. Balikesir Saglik Bil Derg 2012; 1(1): 7-11.
- **Karatas OH, Toy E.** Three-dimensional imaging techniques: A literature review. Eur J Dent 2014; 8(1): 132-140.
- **Kassab NH.** The selection of maxillary anterior teeth width in relation to facial measurements at different types of face form. Al-Rafidain Dent J 2005; 5(1): 15-23.
- **Kern BE.** Anthropometric parameters of tooth selection. J Prosthet Dent 1967; 17(5): 431-437.
- **Kim JY, Lee SJ, Kim TW, Nahm DS, Chang Y.** Classification of the skeletal variation in normal occlusion. Angle orthod 2005; 75(3): 303-311.
- **Kina S, Romanini JC.** Harmonia. Rev Dental Press Estét 2007; 4(2): 67-88, cited by Brandão RCB, Brandão LBC. Finishing procedures in orthodontics: dental dimensions and proportions (microesthetics). Dental Press J Orthod 2013; 18(5): 147-174.
- **Kini AY, Angadi GS.** Biometric ratio in estimating widths of maxillary anterior teeth derived after correlating anthropometric measurements with dental measurements. Gerodontology 2012; 29(2): 674-679.
- **Kokich VO, Kiyak HA, Shapiro PA.** Comparing the perception of dentists and lay people to altered dental esthetics. J Esthet Dent 1999; 11(6): 311-324.

References

- **Konikoff BM, Johnson DC, Schenkein HA, Kwatra N, Waldrop TC.** Clinical crown length of the maxillary anterior teeth pre-orthodontics and post-orthodontics. J Periodontol 2007; 78(4): 645-653.
- **Koralakunte PR, Budihal DH.** A clinical study to evaluate the correlation between maxillary central incisor tooth form and face form in an Indian population. J Oral Sci 2012; (3): 273-278.
- **Ku J, Yang H, Yun K.** A morphometric analysis of maxillary central incisor on the basis of facial appearance in Korea. J Adv Prosthodont 2012; 4(1): 13-17.
- **Kumar MV, Ahila SC, Devi SS.** The science of anterior teeth selection for a completely edentulous patient: a literature review. J Indian Prosthodont Soc 2011; 11: 7-13.
- **Kurkcuoglu A, Bahadıroglu S, Buyukberber Sg, Guclu S, Gurbuz S, Karslıoglu A, Yazıcı C, Pelin C.** Evaluation of lower face heights and ratios according to sex. Rev Arg De Anat Clin 2013; 5(3): 213-221.
- **Kurth JR, Kokich VG.** Open gingival embrasures after orthodontic treatment in adults: prevalence and etiology. Am J Orthod Dentofacial Orthop 2001; 120(2): 116-123.

L

- **Langlois JH, Roggman LA, Casey RJ.** Infant preferences for attractive faces: rudiments of stereotype?. Dev Psychol 1987; 23(3): 363-369.
- **Langlois JH, Roggman LA, Musselman L.** What is average and what is not average about attractive faces?. Psychological Science 1994; 5(4): 214-220.
- **Langlois JH, Ritter JM, Casey RJ, Sawin DB.** Infant attractiveness predicts maternal behaviours and attitudes. Dev Psychol 1995; 31: 464-472.
- **Lavere AM, Marcroft KR, Smith RC, Sarka RJ.** Denture tooth selection: an analysis of the natural maxillary central incisor compared to the length and width of the face. Part I. J Prosthet Dent 1992; 67(5): 661-663.

References

- **Leivesley WD**. The reliability of contour photography for facial measurement. Br J Orthod 1983; 10(1): 34-37.
- **Leong SC, White PS**. A comparison of aesthetic proportions between the oriental and Caucasian nose. Clin Otolaryngol Allied Sci 2004; 29(6): 672-676.
- **Leong SC, White PS**. A comparison of aesthetic proportions between the healthy Caucasian nose and the aesthetic ideal. J Plast Reconstr Aesthet Surg 2006; 59(3): 248-252.
- **Levin EI**. Dental esthetics and golden proportion. J Prosthet Dent 1978; 40(3): 244-252.
- **Lombardi RE**. The principles of visual perception and their clinical application to denture esthetics. J Prosthet Dent 1973; 29(4): 358-382.
- **Lombroso C**. L'AnthropologieCriminelle. Paris: Alcan, 1890: 26-74, cited by Vegter F, Hage JJ. Clinical anthropometry and canons of the face in historical perspective. Plast Reconstr Surg 2000; 106(5): 1090-1096.
- **Lundstrom A**. Tooth size and occlusion in twins. Thesis (Uppsala) Karger, Basle and New York, 1948.
- **Lundstrom A**. Size of teeth and jaws in twins. Br Dent J 1964; 117: 321-326.
- **Lunt Da**. An odotometric study of medieval danes. Acta Odont Scand. 1969, 27:55, cited by Murshid Z, Hashim Ha. Mesiodistal tooth width in a Saudi population: a preliminary report. The Saudi Dental Journal 1993; 5(2): 68-72.

M

- **Maclaren EA, Rifkin R**. Macroesthetics: facial and dentofacial analysis. J Calif Dent Assoc 2002; 30(11): 839-846.
- **Maclaren EA, Tran Coa P**. Smile analysis and esthetic design: "in the zone". Inside Dent 2009; 5(7): 46-48, cited by Maclaren EA, Culp L. smile analysis, the photoshop smile design technique-part 1. J Cosmet Dent 2013; 29(1): 94-108.
- **Maclaren EA, Culp L**. Smile analysis, the photoshop smile design technique-part 1. J Cosmet Dent 2013; 29(1): 94-108.

References

- **Magne P, Belser U.** Bonded porcelain restorations in the anterior dentition: a biomimetic approach. Chicago: Quintessence, 2001; 32: 269-281.
- **Magne P, Gallucci GO, Belser U.** Anatomic crown width/length ratios of unworn and worn maxillary teeth in white subjects. J Prosthet Dent 2003; 89(5): 453-461.
- **Mahadevia S, Daruwala N, Desal S.** Divine orthodontics. JADCH 2011; 1(2): 6-11.
- **Mahesh P, Srinivas Rp, Pavan Kt, Shalini K.** An in vivo clinical study of facial measurements for anterior teeth selection. Aedj 2010; 4(1): 1-6.
- **Mahmood AB.** Facial golden proportions for a sample of Iraqi adults. Iraqi Orthod J 2010; 6(1): 36-38.
- **Mahshid M, Khoshvaghti A, Varshosaz M, Vallaei N.** Evaluation of "golden proportion" in individuals with an esthetic smile. J Esthet Restor Dent 2004; 16(3): 185-192.
- **Malkoç S, Demir A, Uysal T, Canbuldu N.** Angular photogrammetric analysis of the soft tissue facial profile of Turkish adults. Eur J Orthod 2009; 31(2): 174-179.
- **Manera JF, Subtlety JD.** A cephalometric study of the growth of the nose. Am J Orthod 1961; 47(9): 703-705.
- **Marcushamer E, Tsukiyama T, Griffin T, Arguello E, Gallucci G, Magne P.** Anatomical crown width/length ratios of worn and unworn maxillary teeth in Asian subjects. Int J Periodontics Restorative Dent 2011; 31(5): 495-503.
- **Marshall WA, Tanner JM.** Puberty. In: Falkner F, Tanner JM. Human growth. New York: Plenum Publishing 1986; 2: 76-78.
- **Mathes EW, Brennan SM, Haugen PM.** Ratings of physical attractiveness as a function of age. J Soc Psychol 1985; 125(2): 157-168.
- **Matoula S, Panchez H.** Skeletal morphology of attractive and non-attractive faces. The Angle Orthod 2006; 76(2): 204-210.
- **Mavroskoufis F, Ritchie GM.** Variation in size and form between left and right maxillary central teeth. J Prosthet Dent 1980; 43(3): 254-257.

References

- **McCurdy E.** Human proportions. In McCurdy E (Ed.). The notebooks of Leonardo Da Vinci, Vol. 1. London: Reprint Society 1954: 197-204.
- **McDonald F, Ireland AJ.** Diagnosis of the orthodontic patient. New York: Oxford University Press, 1998.
- **McMurrich JP.** Leonardo Da Vinci: the anatomist. baltimore: Williams & Wilkins 1930: 104-110.
- **Meneghini F.** Clinical facial analysis. Springer-Verlag Berlin Heidelberg 2005: 16-17.
- **Meredith G.** Facial photography for orthodontic office. Am J Orthod Dentofac Orthop 1997; 111(5): 463-470.
- **Meredith HW, Chadha IM.** A roentgenographic study of change in head height during childhood and adolescence. J Human Biol 1962; 34(1): 299-319.
- **Michiels LYF, Tourne LPM.** Nasion true vertical: a proposed method of testing the clinical validity of cephalometric measurements applied to a new cephalometric reference line. Int Jr Adult Orthod Orthog Surg 1990; 5(1): 43-52.
- **Milutinovic J, Zelic K, Nedeljkovic N.** Evaluation of facial beauty using anthropometric proportions. J scien world 2014: 8.
- **Mitchell L.** An Introduction to orthodontics. 4th ed. Oxford University Press 2013.
- **Mollov N, Bosio J, Pruszynski J, Wirtz T.** Intra- and inter-examiner reliability of direct facial soft tissue measurements using digital calipers. Journal of the World Federation of Orthodontists 2012; 1(4): 157-161.
- **Morley J, Eubank J.** Macroesthetic elements of smile design. J Am Dent Assoc 2001; 132(1): 39-45.
- **Moyers RE.** Handbook of orthodontics, 4th ed. London, United Kingdom, 1988.
- **Mupparapu M.** Radiation protection guidelines for the practicing orthodontist. Am J Orthod Dentofac Orthop 2005; 128(2): 168-172.

References

- **Muradin MS, Rosenberg A, van der Bilt A, Stoelinga PJ, Koole R**. The reliability of frontal facial photographs to assess changes in nasolabial soft tissues. Int J of Oral Maxillofac Surg 2007; 36(8): 728-734.
- **Murshid Z, Hashim Ha**. Mesiodistal tooth width in a Saudi population: a preliminary report. The Saudi Dental Journal 1993; 5(2): 68-72.
- **Murthy B, Ramani N**. Evaluation of natural smile: golden proportion, RED or Golden percentage. J Conserv Dent 2008; 11(1): 16-21.

N

- **Nahidh M**. The Value of Maxillary Central Incisors and Canines in Gender Determination as an Aid in Forensic Dentistry. Iraqi Dent J 2014; 36(1): 8-12.
- **Naini FB, Gill DS**. Facial aesthetics: 2. clinical assessment. Dent Update 2008; 35(3): 159-170.
- **Naini FB, Moss JP, Gill DS**. The enigma of facial beauty: esthetics, proportions, deformity and controversy. Am J Orthod Dentofac Orthop 2006; 130(3): 277-282.
- **Nanda RS**. The rates of growth of several facial components from serial cephalometric roentgenograms. Am J Orthod 1955; 41(9): 658-673.
- **Nanda RS**. Esthetics and biomechanics in orthodontics. 2nd ed. St. Louis, Mo.: Mosby Elsevier, 2015.
- **Nanda RS, Meng H, Kapila S, Goorhuis J**. Growth changes in the soft tissue facial profile. Angle Orthod 1990; 60(3): 177-190.
- **Naqash T, Bali S**. Evaluation of golden proportion between maxillary anterior teeth in Kashmiri population. IJCCI 2013; 5(2): 3-7.
- **Neger M**. A quantitative method for the evaluation of the soft-tissue facial profile. Am J Orthod 1959; 45(10): 738-751.
- **Nelson SJ**. Weelar's dental anatomy, physiology and occlusion. W.B. Saunders, Philadelphia, 1984: 100.
- **Nikgoo A, Alavi K, Mirfazaelian A**. Assessment of the golden ratio in pleasing smiles. World J Orthod 2009; 10(3): 224-228.

References

- Nithya CS, Ramachandra CS, Shetty PC. Correlation between the apparent widths of the maxillary anteriors and the golden proportion-a survey. J Ind Orthod Soc 2008; 42(3): 9-12.

O

- Ong E, Brown RA, Richmond S. Peer assessment of dental attractiveness. Am J Orthod Dentofacial Orthop 2006; 130(2): 163-169.
- Orozco-Varo A, Arroyo-Cruz G, Martínez-de-Fuentes R, Jiménez-Castellanos E. Biometric analysis of the clinical crown and the width/length ratio in the maxillary anterior region. J Prosthet Dent 2015; 113(6): 565-570.
- Owens EG, Goodacre CJ, Loh PL, Hanke G, Okamura M, Jo KH, Muñoz CA, Naylor WP. A multicenter inter racial study of facial appearance. Part 2: A comparison of intraoral parameters. Int J Prosthodont 2002; 15(3): 283-288.
- Ozdemir ST, Sigirli D, Ercan I, Cankur NS. Photographic facial soft tissue analysis of healthy Turkish young adults: anthropometric measurements. Aesth Plast Surg 2009; 33(2): 175-184.

P

- Park YC, Burstone CJ. Soft tissue profile: fallacies of hard tissue standards in treatment planning. Am J Orthod Dentofac Orthop 1986; 90(1): 52-62.
- Parnia F, Hafezeqoran A, Mahboub F, Moslehifard E, Koodaryan R, Moteyagheni R, Saber F. Proportions of maxillary anterior teeth relative to each other and to golden standard in Tabriz dental faculty students. J Dent Clin Dent 2010; 4(3): 83-86.
- Patel JR, Sethuraman R, Naveen YG, Shah MH. A comparative evaluation of the relationship of inner-canthal distance and inter-alar width to the inter-canine width amongst the Gujarati population. JoAOR 2011; 2(3): 31-38.
- Payne MG. The Reliability of facial soft tissue landmarks with photogrammetry. Master Thesis. Marquette University, 2013.

References

- **Peck H, Peck S**. A concept of facial esthetics. Angle Orthod 1970; 40(4): 284-319.
- **Peck S, Peck L**. Selected aspects of the art and science of facial esthetics. Semin Orthod 1995; 1(2): 105-126.
- **Perrett DI, May KA, Yoshikawa S**. Facial shape and judgments of female attractiveness. Nature 1994; 368(6468): 239-242.
- **Petričević N, Čelebić A, Ibrahimagić-Šeper L, Kovačić I**. Appropriate proportions as guidelines in selection of anterior denture teeth. Medicinski Glasnik 2008; 5(2): 103-108.
- **Phillips C, Greer J, Vig P, Matteson S**. Photocephalometry: errors of projection and landmark location. Am J Orthod 1984; 86(3): 233-243.
- **Pini Np, De-Marchi Lm, Gribel Bf, Ubaldini Alm, Pascotto Rc**. Analysis of the golden proportion and width/height ratios of maxillary anterior dentition in patients with lateral incisor agenesis. J Esthet Restor Dent 2012; 24(6): 402-416.
- **Powell N, Humphreys B**. Proportion of esthetic face. Thieme, New York, 1984: 38.
- **Premkumar S**. Text book of craniofacial growth. Jaypee Bros, 2011.
- **Preston JD**. The golden proportion revisited. J Esthet Dent 1993; 5(6): 247-251.
- **Proffit WR, Fields HW, Ackerman JL**. Contemporary orthodontics. St.Louis: Mosby, 1986.
- **Proffit WR, Fields HW, Sarver DM**. Contemporary orthodontics. 4th ed. St. Louis, Mo.: Mosby Elsevier, 2007.
- **Proffit WR, Fields HW, Sarver DM**. Contemporary orthodontics. 5th Ed. St. Louis: Mosby Elsevier, 2013.
- **Proffit WR, Sarver DM, Ackerman JL**. Orthodontic diagnosis: the development of a problem list. In: Proffit WR, Fields HW, Sarver DM. Contemporary orthodontics. 4th ed. St.Louis: Mosby, 2007; 167-233.

- **Prokopakis EP, Vlastos IM, Picavet V, Trenité GN, Thomas R, Cingi C, Hellings PW.** The golden ratio in facial symmetry. Rhinology 2013; 51(1): 18-21.

R

- **Ramadan OZ.** Relation between photographic facial measurements and lower dental arch measurement in adult Jordanian males with class I normal occlusion. A master thesis, Department of Pedodontics, Orthodontics, and Preventive Dentistry, Collage of Dentistry, University of Mosul, 2000.
- **Raymond E, Pragati A, David W, Darrel G.** The use of anthropometric proportion indices in the measurement of facial attractiveness. Europ J Orthod 2006; 28(3): 274-281.
- **Reyneke JP, Ferretti C.** Clinical assessment of the face. Seminars in Orthodontics 2012; 18(3): 172-186.
- **Rhee SC, Koo SH.** An objective system for measuring facial attractiveness. Plast Reconstr Surg 2007; 119: 1952-1953.
- **Rhodes G, Yoshikawa S, Clark A, Lee K, McKay R, Akamatsu S.** Attractiveness of facial averageness and symmetry in non-western cultures: in search of biologically based standards of beauty. Perception 2001; 30(5): 611-625.
- **Ricketts RM.** The golden divider. J Clin Orthod 1981; 15(11): 752-759.
- **Ricketts RM.** Divine proportion in facial esthetics. Clin Plast Surg 1982**(a)**; 9(4): 401-422.
- **Ricketts RM.** The biologic significance of the divine proportion and Fibonacci series. Am J Orthod 1982**(b)**; 81(5): 351-370.
- **Ricketts RM.** The biologic significance of the divine proportion and Fibonacci series. Am J Orthod 1982**(c)**; 81(5): 351-370.
- **Ricketts RM.** Esthetics, environment, and the law of lip relation. Am J Orthod 1986; 54(4): 272-289.

References

- **Riggio RE, Widaman KF, Tucker JS, Salinas C**. Beauty is more than skin deep: components of attractiveness. Basic and Applied Social Psychology 1991; 12(4): 423-439.
- **Rita ME, Kinga J, Carmen B, Diana C, Horga C, Bögözi B, Alina I**. Aesthetic principles of the upper front teeth: application of golden proportion (levin) and golden percentage (Snow). Acta Medica Marisiensis 2013; 59(1): 25-27.
- **Roberts-Harry D, Sandy J**. Orthodontics. part 2: patient assessment and examination I. BDJ 2003; 195(9): 489-493.
- **Rodríguez CJ**. La antropología forense en la identificación humana. Bogotá, Universidad nacional de Colombia 2004; 48(2): 185-214, cited by Al-Janabi SM. Photogrammetric analysis of facial soft tissue profile of Iraqi adults sample with class I normal occlusion. A master thesis, Department of Orthodontics, University of Baghdad, 2011.
- **Rosenstiel SF**. Dentists' preferences of anterior tooth proportion- a web-based study. J Prosthodont 2000; 9(3): 123-136.
- **Rubenstein AJ, Kalakanis L, Langlois JH**. Infant preferences for attractive faces: a cognitive explanation. Developmental Psychology 1999; 35(3): 848-855.
- **Rufenacht CR**. Principles of esthetic integration. Hanover Park (IL). Quintessence Pub, 2000.

S

- **Sah SK, Zhang HD, Chang T, Dhungana M, Acharya L, Chen LL, Ding YM**. Maxillary anterior teeth dimensions and proportions in a Central Mainland Chinese population. The Chinese journal of dental research 2014; 17(2): 117-124.
- **Sandeep G, Sonia G**. Pattern of dental malocclusion in orthodontic patients in Rwanda: a retrospective hospital based study. Rmj 2012; 69(4): 13-18.
- **Sandler PJ, Murray AM**. Clinical photographs- the gold standard. J Orthod 2002; 29(2): 158-161.

References

- **Sarver DM**. Video cephalometric diagnosis (VCD): A new concept in treatment planning?. Am J Orthod Dentofacial Orthop 1996; 110(2): 128-136.
- **Sarver DM**. Esthetic orthodontics and orthoganthic surgery. St. Louis: CV Mosby, 1997.
- **Sarver DM**. Esthetic orthodontics and orthognathic surgery, St Louis: CV Mosby, 1998.
- **Sarver DM**. Principles of cosmetic dentistry in orthodontics: Part 1. shape and proportionality of anterior teeth. Am J Orthod Dentofac Orthop 2004; 126(6): 749-753.
- **Sarver DM**. Enameloplasty and esthetic finishing in orthodontics: identification and treatment of microesthetic features in orthodontics. Part 1. J Esthet Restor Dent 2011; 23(5): 296-302.
- **Sarver DM, Ackerman MB**. Dynamic smile visualization and quantification: Part 1. evolution of the concept and dynamic records for smile capture. Am J Orthod Dentofac Orthop 2003**(a)**; 124(1): 4-12.
- **Sarver DM, Ackerman MB**. Dynamic smile visualiation and quantification: Part 2. smile analysis and treatment strategies. Am J Orthod Dentofac Orthop 2003**(b)** 124(2): 116-127.
- **Sarver DM, Ackerman MB**. Dynamic smile visualization and quantification and its impact on orthodontic diagnosis and treatment planning. In: The art of smile: integrating Prosthodontics, Orthodontics, Periodontics, Dental Technology and Plastic Surgery. Chicago: Quintessence, 2005: 99-139.
- **Sarver DM, Yanosky M**. Principles of cosmetic dentistry in orthodontics: part 2. Soft tissue laser technology and cosmetic gingival contouring. Am J Orthod Dentofac Orthop 2005; 127(1): 85-90.
- **Sarver DM, Proffit WR, Ackerman JL**. Diagnosis and treatment planning in orthodontics. In: Graber, TM. Vanarsdall, RL. (Eds). Orthodontics: current principles and technique. 3rd ed. Mosby, 2000; 53-54, 88-89.

References

- **Sarwer DB, Grossbart TA, Didie ER.** Beauty and society. Semin Cutan Med Surg 2003; 22(2): 79-92.
- **Saxena S, Thoke B.** 2-D photogrammetry- a new handy diagnostic tool for soft tissue assessment. Orthocj 2012.
- **Scandrett FR, Kerber PE, Umrigar ZR.** A clinical evaluation of techniques to determine the combined width of the maxillary anterior teeth and the maxillary central incisor. J Prosthet Dent 1982; 48(1): 15-22.
- **Seghers MJ, Longacre JJ, Destefano GA.** The golden proportion and beauty. Plast Reconstr Surg 1964; 34(4): 382-386.
- **Sghaireen MG, Al-Zarea BK, Al-Shorman HM, Al-Omiri MK.** Clinical measurement of the height of the interproximal contact area in maxillary anterior teeth. Int J Health Sci (Qassim) 2013; 7(3): 325-330.
- **Sghaireen MG, Albhiran HM, Alzoubi IA, Lynch E, AL-Omiri MK.** Intraoral versus extraoral measurementof the height of the interproximal contact area in maxillary anterior teeth. Med Princ Pract 2015; 24(2): 136-141.
- **Shah SA, Naqash TA, Malik BR.** Effect of Golden proportion evaluation in cosmetic dental restoration of maxillary anterior teeth in Kashmiri population: a research. Medical Science 2014; 10(38): 58-61.
- **Shah SA, Naqash TA, Abdullah S, Bashir U, Gulzar S, Bashir S.** Significance of intercanthal distance in the selection of width of maxillary anterior teeth size in Kashmiri Population: A Research. Int J Health Sci Res 2015; 5(2): 213-216.
- **Shaner DJ, Bamforth JS, Peterson AE, Beattie OB.** Technical note: different techniques, different results-a comparison of photogrammetric and caliper-derived measurements. Am J Phys Anthropol 1998; 106(4): 547-552.
- **Sharma S, Nagpal A, Verma PR.** Correlation between facial measurements and the mesiodistal width of the maxillary anterior teeth. Ijds 2012; 3(4): 20-24.
- **Shetty K, Kumar M, Palagiri K, Amanna S, Shetty S.** Facial measurements as predictors of the length of the maxillary central incisor in a cross section of the

Indian population -a clinical study. Oral Hyg Health 2013; 1: 106. doi: 10. 4172/2332-0702. 1000106.
- **Shetty S, Pitti V, SatishBabu CL, Surendra Kumar GP, Jnanadev KR.** To evaluate the validity of recurring esthetic dental proportion in natural dentition. J Conserv Dent 2011; 14(3): 314-317.
- **Shillingburg HT, Kaplan MJ, Grace CS.** Tooth dimensions. A comparative study. J South Calif Dent Assoc 1972; 40(9): 830-839.
- **Silverman SI.** Physiologic factors in complete denture esthetics. Dent clin North Am 1967: 115-122.
- **Sinavarat P, Anunmana C, Hossain S.** The relationship of maxillary canines to the facial anatomical landmarks in a group of Thai people. J Adv Prosthodont 2013; 5(4): 369-373.
- **Sinclair PM.** The divine proportion. Am J Orthod 1982; 82: 166-167.
- **Sitthiphan P, Viwattanatipa N, Amornvit P, Shrestha B, Srithavaj MT, Alam MK.** Comparison of maxillary anterior teeth crown ratio (width/length) between gender in Laotian population. International Medical Journal 2015; 22(3): 199-205.
- **Smith, Stevenson, Simpson, William K.** The art and architecture of ancient Egypt, 3rd ed. Yale University Press (Penguin/Yale History of Art), 1998, ISBN 0300077475.
- **Snijder GAS.** Het ontstaan van den proportie-kanonbij de grieken. Utrecht, The Netherlands: Oosthoek, 1928; 5-41, cited by Vegter F, Hage JJ. Clinical anthropometry and canons of the face in historical perspective. Plast Reconstr Surg 2000; 106(5): 1090-1096.
- **Snow SR.** Esthetic smile analysis of anterior tooth width: the golden percentage. J Esthet Dent 1999; 11(4): 177-184.
- **Stappert CFJ, Tarnow DP, Chu SJ.** Proximal contact areas of the maxillary anterior dentition. Int J Periodontics Restorative Dent 2010; 30(5): 471-477.

References

- **Stephan CN, Henneberg M, Sampson W**. Predicting nose projection and pronasale position in facial approximation: A test of published methods and proposal of new guidelines. Am J Phys Anthropol 2003; 122(3): 240-250.
- **Sterrett JD, Oliver T, Robinson F, Fortson W, Knaak B, Russell CM**. Width/length ratios of normal clinical crowns of the maxillary anterior dentition in man. J Clin Periodontol 1999; 26(3): 153-157.
- **Stoner M**. A photogrammetric analysis of the facial profile. Am J Orthod 1955; 41(6): 453-469.
- **Strajnic L, Vuletic I, Vucinic P**. The significance of biometric parameters in determining anterior teeth width. Vojnosanit Pregl 2013; 70(7): 653-659.
- **Subtelny JD**. Longitudinal study of soft tissue facial structures and their profile characteristics, defined in relation to underlying skeletal structure. Am J Orthod 1959; 45: 481-507.
- **Sulaiman E, Yaakub Ms, Zulkifli Na, Abdullah M, Gonzalez Mag**. Existence of golden proportion in maxillary anterior teeth of university of Malaya dental students. Annal Dent Univ Malaya 2010; 17: 9-14.
- **Swaddle JP, Cuthill IC**. Asymmetry and human facial attractiveness: symmetry may not always be beautiful. Proc Biol Sci 1995; 261(1360): 111-116.
- **Sweirgenga D, Oeserle LJ, Messersmith ML**. Cephalometric values for adults Mexican. Am J Orthod Dentofac Orthop 1994; 106(2): 146-155.

T

- **Tarnow DP, Magner AW, Fletcher P**. The effect of distance from the contact point to the crest bone of the presence or absence of the interproximal dental papilla. J Periodontol 1992; 68(12): 995-996.
- **Terry RI, Davis JS**. Components of facial attractivness. Percept Mot Skills 1976; 42: 918-934.
- **Thornhill R, Gangestad SW**. Facial attractiveness. Trends in Cognitive Sciences 1999; 3(12): 452-460.

- **Touati BT**. Defining form and position. Pract Periodontics Aesthet Dent 1998; 10(7): 800, 802-803.
- **Trpkova B, Major P, Prasad N, Nebbe B**. Cephalometric landmarks identification and reproducibility: a meta-analysis. Am J Orthod and Dentofacial Orthop 1997; 112: 165-170.

U

- **Umer F, Khan FR, Khan A**. Golden proportion in visual dental smile in Pakistani population: a pilot study. Acta Stomatol Croat. 2010; 44(3): 168-175.
- **Urdang L**. The random house dictionary of the English language. New York, random house, 1968: 985.

V

- **Vadavadagi SV, Hombesh MN, Choudhury GK, Deshpande S, Anusha CV, Murthy DK**. Variation in size and form between left and right maxillary central incisor teeth. J Int Oral Health 2015; 7(2): 33-36.
- **Van Teijlingen E, Hundley V**. The importance of pilot studies. Nurs Stand 2002; 16(40): 33-36.
- **Varjao FM, Nogueira SS**. Nasal width as a guide for the selection of maxillary complete denture anterior teeth in four racial groups. Prosthodontics J 2006; 15(6): 353-358.
- **Varjão FM, Nogueira SS, Russi S, ArioliFilho JN**. Correlation between maxillary central incisor form and face form in 4 racial groups. Quintessence Int 2006; 37(10): 767-771.
- **Vegter F, Hage JJ**. Clinical anthropometry and canons of the face in historical perspective. Plast Reconstr Surg 2000; 106(5): 1090-1096.

References

- **Verma KC, Puri V, Sharma TC**. Anthropometric study of inner canthal, interpupillary and outer orbital dimensions - range of normal. Indian Pediatr 1978; 15: 349-352.
- **Vig PS, Cohen AM**. Vertical growth of the lips: a serial cephalometric study. Am J Orthod 1979; 75(4): 405-415.

- **Ward DH**. Proportional smile design using the recurring esthetic dental (RED) proportion. Dent Clin North Am 2001; 45(1): 143-154.
- **Ward DH**. A study of dentists' preferred maxillary anterior tooth width proportions: comparing the recurring esthetic dental proportion to other mathematical and naturally occurring proportions. J Esthet Restor Dent 2007; 19(6): 324-339.
- **Ward DH**. Using the RED proportion to engineer the perfect smile. Dent Today 2008; 27(5): 114-117.
- **Weeden J, Sabini J**. Physical attractiveness and health in western societies: a review. Psychological Bulletin by the American Psychological Association, 2005; 131(5): 635-653.
- **Wehner PJ, Hickey JC, Boucher CO**. Selection of artificial teeth. J Prosthet Dent 1967; 18(3): 222-232.
- **Williams RP, Rinchuse AD, Zullo TG**. Perceptions of midline deviations among different facial types. Am J Orthod Dentofacial Orthop 2014; 145(2): 249-255.
- **Wolfart S, Menzel H, Kern M**. Inability to relate tooth forms to face shape and gender. Eur J Oral Sci 2004; 112(6): 471-476.
- **Wolfart S, Thormann H, Freitag S, Kern M**. Assessment of dental appearance following changes in incisor proportions. Eur J Oral Sci 2005; 113(2): 159-165.

References

Z

- **Zarb GA, Bolender CL, Hickey JC, Carlson GE**. Bouchers prosthodontic treatment for edentulous mouth. 10th ed. St Louis: The C.V. Mosby Co, 1990: 3-27.
- **Zlataric DK, Kristek E, Celebic A**. Analysis of width/length ratios of normal clinical crowns of the maxillary anterior dentition: correlation between dental proportions and facial measurements. Int J Prosthodont 2007; 20: 313-315.

Appendix I

The consent form that used in the study:

College of dentistry

University of Baghdad

This Informed Consent Form is for males and females who are students at University of Baghdad, and who I am inviting to participate in research. The title of my research project is photographic analysis of macro and micro-aesthetic appearance in a sample of Iraqi adults with class I normal occlusion.

Dana Rifat Mohammed

Orthodontic Department/College of Dentistry/ University of Baghdad

*Information:

I am an orthodontic postgraduate student at Dentistry College/University of Baghdad. I am doing my research on macro- and micro-aesthetic appearance which are an important divisions of aesthetics in orthodontics, I am going to give you information and invite you to be part of this research. This research will involve a single extra and intraoral frontal photograph for each participant, your participation in this research is entirely voluntary. It is your choice whether to participate or not. The information that we collect from this research project will be kept confidential. Information about you that will be collected during the research will be put away and only the researchers will be able to see it. Any information about you will have a number on it instead of your name.

*Certificate of Consent:

I have read the foregoing information. I consent voluntarily to participate as a participant in this research.

Name of Participant   Signature of Participant

Date

Appendix II

The case sheet that used in the study:
Name:……………………… Age:…………….. Gender:…………
Date:………………… Tel. No.: …………. Case No.: ………..
Past Medical History: ………………………………………………………………
Past Dental History: ……………………………………………………………....

Clinical Examination:

1-Skeletal Examination

-Anteroposterior Relation: …………

-Vertical relation: …………..

- Horizontal Relation: …………….

2-Dental Examination

-Number of teeth:

7	6	5	4	3	2	1	1	2	3	4	5	6	7
7	6	5	4	3	2	1	1	2	3	4	5	6	7

-Molar Classification: ClassI….   Right…. Left….

-Canine Classification: ClassI….   Right… Left….

-Incisors Classification: ClassI…   Right… Left….

-Overjet….mm.   Overbite…..mm.

-Crossbite: Present…… Absent…..

-Habits: ……   Digit sucking….. Mouth breathing….. lip sucking….. Nail biting……

-Oral hygien: good…. Fair…. Poor….   Periodontal status: good…. Fair….. poor…..

-Dental deformities or anomalies: Present…… Absent……